"Sinful" Acts, Sexual Orientation, And Religious Indoctrination:

Unraveling the Neuroanatomical, Neurophysiological, and Neurochemical Aberrancies

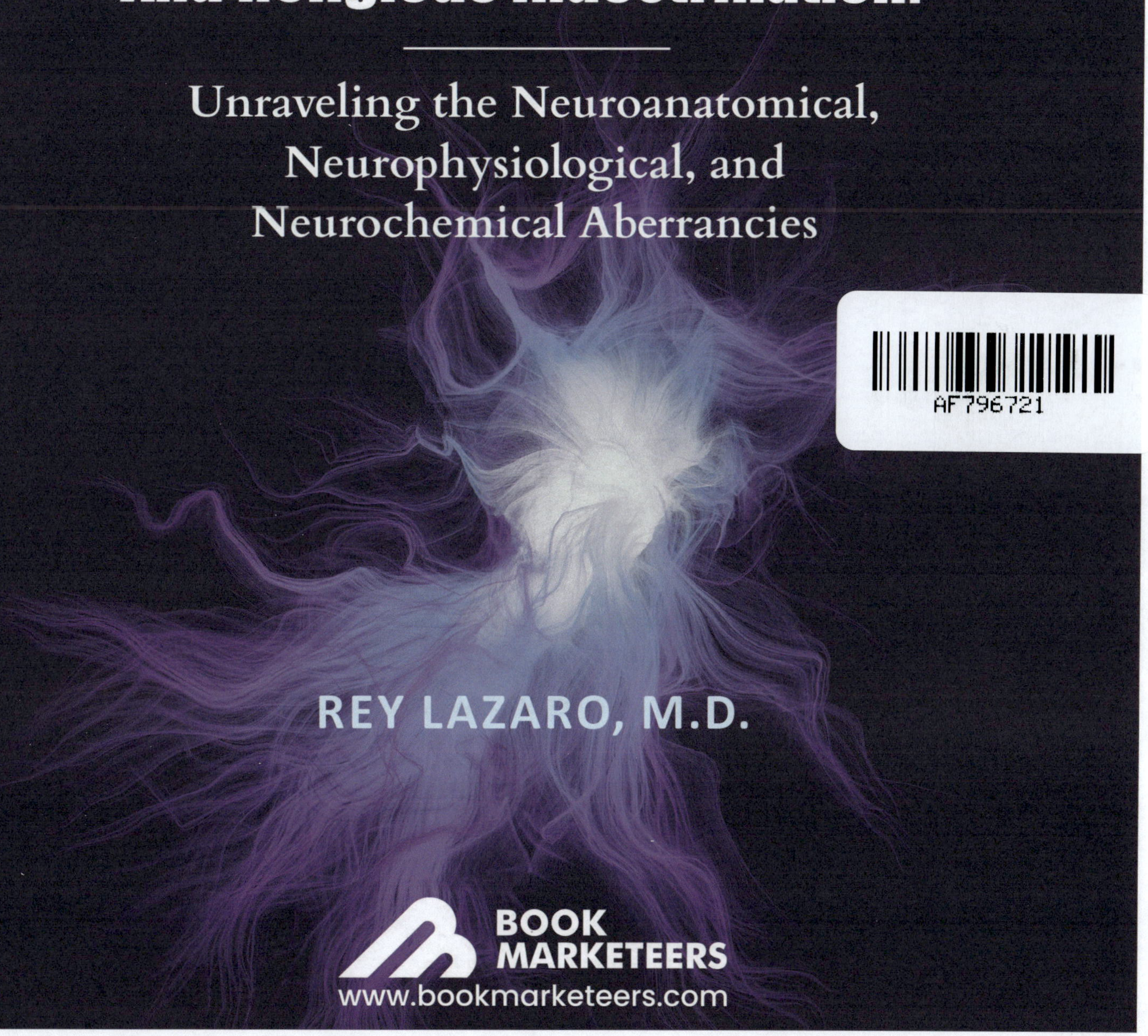

REY LAZARO, M.D.

BOOK MARKETEERS
www.bookmarketeers.com

Also written by Rey Lazaro, M.D.

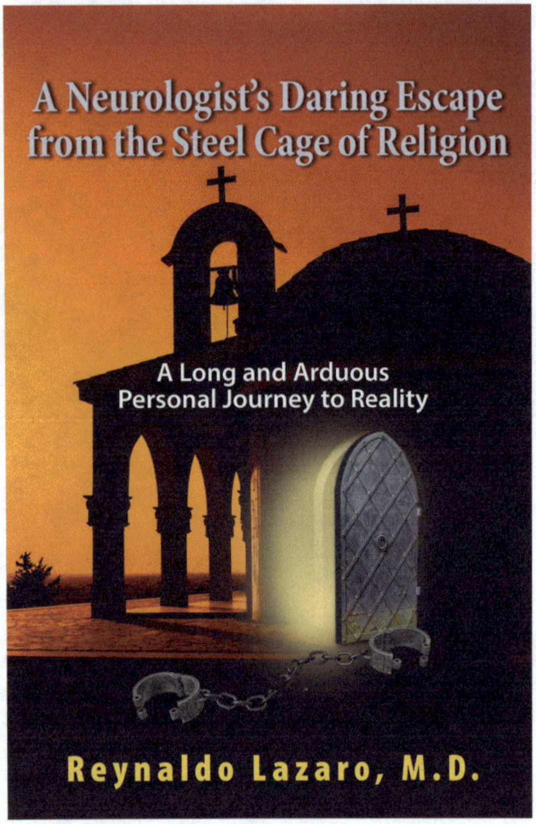

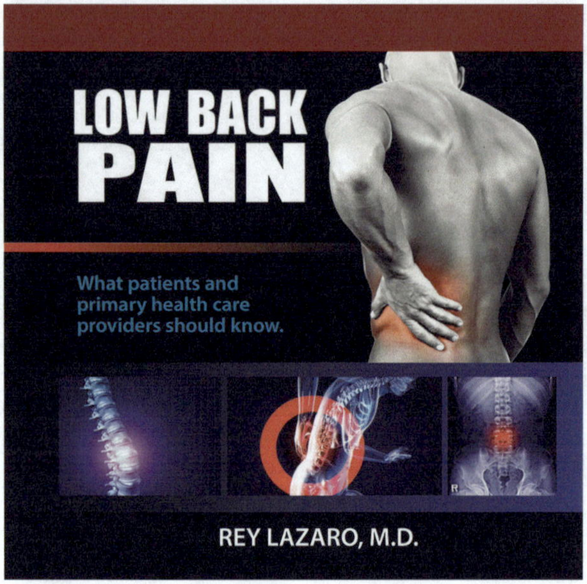

 ISBN: Number Printed in the United States of America Published by: Bookmarketeers.com

Edited by Sribendi, Ontario, Canada. Art works provided by Maa Illustrations, art@maaillustrations.com. Graphic design by Elizabeth Parry.

ISBN: 978-1-962905-30-5
Library of Congress: 2023901073
Printed: January 2023

DEDICATION

This work is dedicated to all freethinkers, truth seekers, conservatives, progressives, libertarians, atheists, agnostics, physicians, and health care professionals. It was written to provide, in scientific terms, explanations of why some people commit acts that go against moral and legal principles, and why some people develop certain sexual orientations and personalities that border the mainstream. It is NOT meant to mitigate the accountability and culpability for those acts that are considered immoral or illegal by modern-day society.

This dedication is extended to my religious classmates (medical class of 1970) and immediate members of my family—most of whom I have offended on various occasions—whose faith was permanently cemented in their limbic systems during childhood, when they did not have the ability to distinguish between beliefs and facts or before their reasoning skills had a chance to develop.

"A rigidly traditional individual's perceptivity, like that of a captive frog in a deep well, is able to function only within narrow parameters. He does not realize that there are boundless vistas of knowledge beyond the scope of the well, therefore, his mental and intellectual evolution remains stunted. He is unable to take advantage of the knowledge available beyond his limited horizon." – **Ahmad as-Sowayyan. The Dangers of Narrow-Mindedness – kallamullah.com/personality12.html**

"When I do good, I feel good. When I do bad, I feel bad. That's my religion." – **Abraham Lincoln (1809-1865) – 16th president of the US, American lawyer, and statesman**

"My country is the world, and my religion is to do good." – Thomas Paine (1737-1809) – **American political activist and philosopher**

"Freethinkers are those who are willing to use their mind without prejudice and without fearing to understand things that clash with their own customs, privileges, or beliefs. This state of mind is not common but it is essential for right thinking." – **Leo Tolstoy (1828-1910) – Russian author, On Life and Essays on Religion**

"The very concept of sin comes from the Bible. Christianity offers to solve a problem of its own making! Would you be thankful to a person who cut you with a knife in order to sell you a bandage?" – **Dan Barker in Godless: How an Evangelical Preacher became one of America's Leading Atheists**

"The difference between a miracle and a fact is exactly the difference between a mermaid and a seal." – **Mark Twain (1835-1910), American writer humorist, publisher, and lecturer**

"Many religious people are kind, loving and good. Many are not. Whether it is the belief system that molds them or their nature, it is hard to say. Most are woefully misinformed and underexposed to material that could change them for the better. But literacy takes reading, change takes effort and enlightenment takes courage. In the end, "Ye shall know the truth, and the truth shall make you free" (John 8:32) – **Tim C. Leedom, editor, The Book Your Church Doesn't Want You to Read**

"The way to see by faith is to shut the eye of reason" – Benjamin Franklin (1706-1790) – **American author, Founding Father, political theorist, and diplomat**

PREFACE

Have you ever wondered why some humans are susceptible to infection, react differently or adversely to the actions or side effects of some drugs, metabolize foods at a different rate, are prone to allergic reactions, or are likely to develop various disorders that affect the internal organs? Science has taught us that these differences are related to the innate genetic makeup of the individual, together with biochemical and metabolic alterations that place the individual at risk for developing certain diseases. Psychologically, why do humans behave differently? Some are shy, calm, mild-mannered, carefree, self-assertive, confident, composed, anxious, easily depressed, audacious, passionate, flamboyant, boisterous, hyperactive, overly aggressive, hostile, or temperamental. Some are sexually aggressive, while others are prone to rage and violence and are likely to commit crimes or sinful acts. Science has revealed that part of the brain, called the limbic system, determines personality and regulates the behavior of mammals.

Why do people become Christians, Jews, Muslims, or Buddhists, or choose to join other religious organizations and tenaciously adhere to their teachings and beliefs? Why do some people choose to become nonbelievers, agnostics, or atheists. Today, hundreds of millions of nonbelievers exist worldwide, most of them residing in Asian countries (China, India, Japan, Vietnam, and South Korea), while others live in Europe (Russia, Germany, France, the United Kingdom, and Ukraine). Those Asian countries that escaped direct annexation by the Spanish empire never received any form of teachings about Christian beliefs and doctrines. However, it's a different situation in the Philippines, an island nation in Southeast Asia, where the practice of Christianity (Catholicism) is fervent and widespread—the result of 400 years of Spanish colonization. The fact that the Philippines is the only predominantly Catholic nation in Asia is a living testament to oppressive religious indoctrination—a teaching process used by the Spaniards to groom the naïve and innocent mind of the Filipinos. The same process was used by Christopher Columbus and his missionaries to force the American natives to convert to Christianity. Thousands of natives, who were called "heathens," were murdered when they refused to do so.

Why do some people develop different sexual orientations or sexual perversions? Are you aware that homosexuals were punished or even put to death by religious authorities during ancient times? Clergy sexual abuse of minors is a global and serious concern among all members of society, both past and present. Have you ever asked yourself how many priests who became canonized saints many years ago were pedophiles? We probably will never know the true story, but one thing is clear: there was no public scrutiny of the Catholic church, and there were no media reporters and whistle blowers to expose the perverted misdeeds of powerful clergies during that time—had there been, they would have suffered severe repercussions. I understand that these questions will hit a raw nerve among devout believers, but these are practical questions, and inquiring minds want to know the answers. Is pedophilia a brain disorder? According to divine laws and the present legal system, this behavior is unquestionably punishable. What if a pedophile has an abnormal limbic system and orbitofrontal cortex? Are sinful acts manifestations of anatomical, physiological, and chemical aberrancies in the brain or simply natural behavior of humans? If they are manifestations of an abnormal brain and are punishable at the same time, will people with abnormal hearts, livers, lungs, kidneys, stomachs, and intestines, for no fault of their own, be punished too?

All organs consist of tissues derived from embryonic stem cells. Basically, they have a similar genetic makeup to that of the zygote, a diploid cell that results from the union between the male (spermatozoon) and female (ovum) reproductive cells. During the complex process of maturation, the stem cells of the zygote migrate, proliferate, and conglomerate to form organs, and then begin to execute the functions they are destined to do. The heart pumps blood, including oxygen that the lungs absorb in the alveoli. The blood distributes oxygen and combats infection, the abdominal organs convert foods to energy, the kidneys and large intestines eliminate excess byproducts of metabolism, and the brain is responsible for defining our personality. It is the seat of higher intellectual function. It perceives sensory stimuli and controls and integrates locomotion, in concert with the musculoskeletal system, which consists of muscles, tendons, bones, joints, ligaments, and cartilages. Therefore, despite the molecular similarities in the genetic framework, cells function in many different ways depending on the organs they are part of.

The differences in a person's behavior depend on how the individual perceives a certain incoming stimulus from within or outside the body. Regardless of race, color, religion, or sexual orientation, each and every one of us acts in a certain manner to express our intentions and desires—and those actions are dictated by the intricate and complex neural network within our brain. This network is located in the limbic system of the brain, a C-shaped region within the cerebral hemispheres extending from the frontal, temporal, and parietal lobes. This system is connected directly and indirectly to all parts of the body. The emotions that humans and animals display are the result of stimuli originating from all parts of the body and relayed via the nerve fiber tracts of the spinal cord, brainstem, and visual, auditory, and olfactory systems. A stimulus reaches the limbic system, where it is processed and interpreted as pleasant or unpleasant, good or bad. The emotional reactions induced by the stimulus can vary. The individual may become happy or sad, calm or angry, fearful or fearless, composed or violent; all of these responses are mediated by numerous chemical neurotransmitters stored in and released from the synapses of the neural network of the limbic system.

A passionate and violent reaction that results in serious injury or the death of an individual is considered sinful and illegal by all members of society. Religious people will label this reaction as evil, but some professionals and scientists will label it as a reflection of the heightened physiological and chemical activities of pools of interconnecting neurons in the limbic system and cerebrum. This is how the battle between belief system and science continues; the former use hearsay to make an argument and the latter use observation, logic, and experimentation to make and establish a point. Both factions run parallel to each other, with no apparent chance of converging.

A well-established fact is that human behavior can be altered or modified by the administration of drugs or medications that either excite or inhibit the actions of various neurotransmitters. Similarly, behavior can be altered by certain disease processes, such as circulatory disturbances, tumors, autoimmune disorders, infection, and trauma, by epigenetic mechanisms, and by several environmental and nutritional factors. These conditions can stimulate or irritate various cerebral centers and may produce hallucinatory or illusory phenomena, including "out of body" experiences (literally, one's self leaving the physical body) and "near-death" experiences. These phenomena were quite likely experienced by the ancients and could have been the basis of beliefs in the existence of the soul—an imaginary and dubious entity whose presumed final destiny, in simplistic terms, is either heaven (if the person is good) or hell (if the person is bad).

While I was writing the book titled, A *Neurologist's Daring Escape from the Steel Cage of Religion: A Long and Arduous Personal Journey to Reality*, and while working on the present book, I came to the realization that educating children based on belief and hearsay without objective evidence is wrongful. I am in full agreement with freethinkers and truth seekers who believe that, as children grow up, they should be allowed to ask questions and be encouraged to think independently and formulate their own judgments. I also became convinced that my religious classmates' religiosity (some are really hyperreligious) is a form of obsessive–compulsive behavior.

In addition to religious education instilled into the brains of believers during childhood, another major reason why believers are pertinacious in their beliefs is a lack of understanding of the mechanisms of how the brain works. Perhaps they should all receive an easy-to-understand course in neuroanatomy, neurochemistry, neurophysiology, neuropathology, and genetics. Realistically and logistically, this can be difficult to accomplish, especially in people who have had a permanent set of beliefs instilled into their limbic system during childhood. Moreover, the intellectual differences that exist among humans—professionals and nonprofessionals alike—will pose an additional hindrance to this type of learning system. I am not implying that religious people have lower intellect; however, when an indoctrination process succeeds during childhood, the information stored in the limbic system is almost always permanent, and that's regrettable. It can certainly interfere with the rational thinking process.

Luckily for me, I did not fall victim to such a process, so I was able to free myself from the powerful grip of religion. My inquiring mind led me to set aside the belief system, and instead explore the many inconsistencies, contradictions, hypocrisies, ironies, and paradoxes that plague the practice of religion. Believers should study the other side of their belief systems, analyze and take a close look at the opposing views, be percipient and open-minded, and formulate sound judgments. In this modern, technologically sophisticated society, where everything is fact-checked, it is ironic that the same people who continue to hold onto their fixated and stagnant belief systems are the same people who take advantage of and benefit from the numerous advances in science. They pray to an invisible supernatural being up in the sky and ask for blessings and forgiveness and to be "saved," and yet they rely on science to meet and satisfy their daily needs. Does this fit the definition of "double standard?"

Is the practice of religion a "forme fruste" (not so typical or partial form of a disease) of obsessive-compulsive disorder (OCD)? Is hyperreligiosity a form of mental illness? OCD is defined as an anxiety-driven condition characterized by repetitive behaviors that place a person at the mercy of uncontrollable thoughts. Religious people have the compulsion to go to church and are fearful that a failure to do so is a sin and may make their God angry. The emotion of fear, especially the fear of eternal punishment, is stored in the amygdala and the entire limbic system. The urge to believe in an invisible deity becomes instinctively overwhelming. Believers react sternly and harshly (or even commit mass murders) when their beliefs are challenged. They argue with nonbelievers by pointing to the miracles, apparitions, and mind-control verses described and written in the Bible. They tend to develop a superiority complex because of their mindset that God is on their side, is present in all corners of the world, and monitors all activities human beings do every day, every hour, every minute, every second, every millisecond, and every microsecond. Most believers offer prayers for nonbelievers to "save" them from going to hell. This is a kind and generous, but scientifically naïve, gesture on their part. Believers have the mentality and strong conviction that all good deeds must be contingent upon belief in God to guarantee a place in heaven. Personally, however, I find it difficult to be beholden to them for their generous deeds, since I do not amalgamate good deeds with belief in the supernatural. I do not subscribe to that religious cliché—"be good and be saved." I do my best to be good because that is the right thing to do. Abraham Lincoln, the 16th president of the U.S., remarked, "When I do good, I feel good. When I do bad, I feel bad. That's my religion."

Do believers have abnormal regulatory interactions between their inhibitory and excitatory neurotransmitters? The believers' passion and commitment to the never-been-seen supernatural being they believe exists are strangely astonishing. Religious practices, especially among Catholics, are so routine and predictable. Before entering the church, congregants dip their index and third fingers into "holy water" (likely contaminated with various microorganisms) contained in a small vessel (called a stoup) that has been blessed by a member of the clergy, and they then make the sign of a cross with those wet fingers. After a confession, the confessor (who, incidentally, may be a sinner himself) administers a penance to the penitent; this usually consists of reciting several prayers many times, including praying the rosary. Mass and faith-based sermons are methodical and rhythmical. Congregants kneel, sit, and stand in unison each time the priest proceeds to another segment of the mass. They sing the same emotionally charged songs and recite the same prayers over and over again. Communion (a round, thin piece of white bread) is given to recipients either on the tongue or on the hand, while the priest utters a phrase, "The body of Christ." Then they sip a small amount of wine, which represents the "blood" of Christ. Nobody knows how this practice originated but it can be easily interpreted as a form of ritual cannibalism. At the conclusion of the mass, congregants feel refreshed and relieved that their sins are presumably forgiven, so to speak. This pleasant feeling resembles the sensation that drug or alcohol addicts experience when the addictive substance is reintroduced into the body at the time when its effect begins to wane.

Interestingly, prayers to God have never prevented natural disasters, war, deaths, famine, or microbial pandemics. Believers predictably always use these two words "God's will" to explain why these unavoidable catastrophes and tragedies in life have been recurring for eons, despite their prayers. The recent COVID pandemic resulted in millions of deaths, various complications from the virus and vaccines, worldwide political mud-slinging, academic learning setbacks for children, and economic downturn. Climate change continues to divide people politically, as oil-producing nations continue to rake in huge profits and, at the same time, choke the finances of the general public. Hurricanes in Florida have resulted in billions in property damage, miseries among the citizens, and many deaths. Several countries, such as Russia, Communist China, North Korea, and Iran, continue to intimidate their neighboring countries and the West.

God, do you love us? If you do, why do you allow all these things to happen? Humans have not seen you or the "Holy Spirit" for thousands of years, not since Jesus Christ, your "son," died on the cross for the "sins" of humanity. You did not prevent the two world wars, which resulted in the loss of millions and millions of innocent lives and enormous property damage. Did you send the souls of those who committed war crimes, including Hitler, to hell? If you did, will you please show us the evidence.

Bill Maher, an American TV personality, remarked, "Religion is a neurological disorder. I don't ridicule religion. It ridicules itself." Is there a relationship between religious indoctrination, obsessive-compulsive behavior, addiction, and the dopamine reward system? The answer is a resounding YES!!! Dopamine is a well-known neurotransmitter because of its relation to Parkinson's Disease (PD), a movement disorder characterized pathologically by degeneration of the neurons that produce dopamine. These neurons are located in the substantia nigra and ventral tegmental area of the midbrain and in the hypothalamus. Dopamine is also synthesized in the peripheral nervous system. Apart from its role in PD, dopamine plays a major role in several body functions, such as memory, movements, mood, attention, cognition, motivation, behavior, and pleasurable rewards. It also mediates drug addiction, a particular condition that can be difficult to control. Addiction is a chronic and relapsing disease characterized by drug-induced, compulsive seeking behavior or craving for drugs. The craving is mediated by dopamine, which is released when a person experiences a pleasant sensation due to stimulation of the pathways of the reward system in the nucleus accumbens, a structure located below the anterior limb of the internal capsule and anterior to the anterior commissure (Figure 1). Most laypeople find it easy to tell an addicted person to simply give up the addiction and "get over it." If that person is unable to overcome the habit, the laypeople will often say, "that person is hopeless and simply lacks willpower." Obviously, overcoming addiction is easier said than done. Science has confirmed how hard it can be for the addicted to end their habits because of the changes that occur in brain chemistry in addiction. Drugs such as marijuana, heroin, amphetamines, and cocaine have been known to mimic the action of endogenous neurotransmitters or to prevent their natural release and re-uptake activities in the neuronal synapses. To make matters worse, some drugs, even marijuana, can induce violent behavior and psychosis and result in criminal acts.

Pleasurable experiences, such as sex, delicious foods, feeling "high" from alcohol or drugs, and winning huge sums of money from gambling or the lottery, are mediated by the pleasure system located in the dopaminergic system of the nucleus accumbens and mesolimbic pathway. Just like drug-seeking, religion is a learned behavior resulting from repeated indoctrination and nurturing. In the long run, it sets the stage for complex interactions among dopaminergic, glutaminergic, and GABAergic activities in the striatum and the limbic system. Pleasure derived from praying together, with religion priming and interacting with the dopamine pleasure system, forms the basis for obsessive-compulsive behavior among the religiously indoctrinated.

TABLE OF CONTENTS

INTRODUCTION

"The deepest sin against the human mind is to believe things without evidence" – **Aldous Huxley (1894-1963) – English writer and philosopher**

"To compel a man to furnish funds for the propagation of ideas he disbelieves and abhors is sinful and tyrannical." – **Thomas Jefferson (1743-1826), 3rd president of the United States**

"Science is the poetry of reality." – **Richard Dawkins, Author of the God Delusion**

"All religions are equally sublime to the ignorant, useful to the politicians, and ridiculous to the philosophers." – **Lucretius (94 BC – 49 BC)**

"The problem with writing about religion is that you run the risk of offending sincerely religious people, and they come after you with machetes." – **Dave Barry, American author, columnist, humorist**

"You don't need religion to have morals. If you can't determine right from wrong then you lack empathy, not religion." – **Funny God Fearing Saying (www.geckoandfly.com)**

Sin is defined as an immoral act that is considered a transgression against divine law. It is a failure to do what is perceived to be right according to a person's religion and societal culture. The word sin is derived from the Old English "synn," which means moral wrongdoing, mischief, guilt, misdeed, or offense against God. The definition is basically spiritual, but it turns a blind eye to the fact that every action man does is controlled and regulated by various pools of interconnecting neurons in the limbic system of the brain—the inner part of the brain that mediates behavior and determines the personality of all beings, including humans and lower forms of animals. When these neural interconnections are modulated by family upbringing and social influence or altered and disrupted by various disease processes, constellations of mental symptoms and behavioral disturbances invariably occur.

A person suffering from borderline personality or psychotic disorder may commit acts that are considered by many to be objectionable and sinful. A homeless paranoid schizophrenic dwelling in the subway tunnels of New York City may commit murder while actively hallucinating and hearing voices urging him to kill a bystander. Killing, unequivocally, is a mortal sin according to the Christian religion. So, where will the soul of that schizophrenic go when he dies—hell or heaven? In the court of law, his act is a crime but, by reason of insanity, that person is likely to be exonerated. That outcome will certainly infuriate the relatives of the victim, even with the understanding that there is a scientific basis for the act. Killing is always condemned by all sectors of society, and it is regrettable and unfortunate when committed by a mentally deranged person. Some people suffering from psychosis are sometimes ridiculed and treated differently by the poorly informed and less educated members of society.

"Thou shalt not kill." Did God specify to Moses what was meant by the sixth commandment? Were there any exceptions? Obviously, in those days, medical science did not exist, and nobody knew how to recognize the symptoms of psychiatric and neurological diseases, such as paranoid schizophrenia, chronic posttraumatic encephalopathy, brain tumors, infection, and other neurodegenerative disorders. How many people were executed as a result of those mental conditions in ancient times?

People who committed mass murders and atrocities have existed since our ape-man ancestors and modern hominids began to roam the Earth. Quite possibly, some of them might have suffered from central nervous system disorders that drove them to commit heinous acts. The likes of Adolf Hitler, Augusto Pinochet, Joseph Stalin, Osama Bin Laden, Pol Pot, Saddam Hussein, Ferdinand Marcos, and other dictators, most lately Vladimir Putin, might have harbored neurons in their limbic lobes that were "abnormally wired and misconnected" from each other—to put it in a superficial way. These abnormal neurons communicate with each other but "misuse" the neurotransmitters released from their synapses, resulting in a loss of rationality, compassion, and sympathy toward fellow human beings. Similarly, children who grow up without proper parental supervision and education and those who grow up in a dysfunctional family whose members are either alcoholics or drug abusers, or both, are more than likely to develop improperly connected neurons. The result is an inability to recognize what is good and bad, or what is right and wrong. This is exactly what is happening in some urban cities, where the crime rate is high and where children grow up unsupervised. They enter and live in a violent society with no concept of responsibility and accountability for their actions or respect for others' lives. Where will their souls go when they die?

Religious tutelage, consisting of belief in God, heaven, hell, daily prayers, confession, and communion, is a routine and compulsory education that religious adults inculcate into the immature mind of a growing child. It is also called indoctrination or, colloquially, brainwashing. Although these two terms are generally considered distinct from each other, they share one common denominator—grooming and molding the mind through repeated inculcation of a belief system or ideology. The process may eventually make the child treat his peers with indifference if they belong to other religions. Parents teach their children to believe in a powerful but invisible being, and that a child's failure to do so will result in eternal torture. That invisible being must be praised and adored at all times, or the child will pay the consequences. According to agnostics and atheists, educating children in this manner before they reach the age of reason is unjustified, and strictly speaking, can be considered a form of child abuse. It creates feelings of guilt, fear, and anxiety and generates obsessive-compulsive behavior that almost always persists throughout the child's lifetime. James Watson, Nobel Prize-winning biologist and geneticist, remarked, "The luckiest thing that ever happened to me was that my father didn't believe in God, and so he had no hang-ups about souls. I see ourselves as products of evolution, which itself is a great mystery."

In religious and legal terms, killing fellow human beings is simply wrong. This is a basic tenet of a civilized society, but life is full of contradictions. Those who are religious know full well that the God of the Old Testament—a merciless Middle Eastern tyrant who "created" the great global flood that killed thousands and thousands of people—is wrathful, cruel, misogynistic, racist, genocidal, mean, homophobic, jealous, vengeful, outrageous, inflexible, and prejudiced. Inexplicably, the God of the New Testament is exactly the opposite—loving, just, kind, merciful, and full of grace. Are these two Gods the same? They obviously appear different, but to devout religious scholars and believers, they are the same, and there is only one God, claimed to be immutable and inseparable. To the critics, the God of the Old Testament and the God of the New Testament are divergent and incongruous, no matter how the faithful spin the issue. It is unfathomable how the two Gods, who ruled the universe separately hundreds (?) or even thousands (?) of years apart, can be considered one and the same. Of course, nobody is allowed to question this issue, for fear of being accused of blasphemy and going to hell—the mindset cemented in the limbic system of the indoctrinated.

As a nonbeliever in the existence of soul or spirit, I was inspired by my deeply religious classmates' negative regard of me to write this book and to present sinful acts from a different angle and perspective. The inspiration grew deeper after I became quite convinced that my colleagues' limited knowledge of neuroanatomy, neurophysiology, neuropathology and neurochemistry is partly responsible for their anachronistic views and pertinacity in religious beliefs that were inculcated into their limbic systems by their parents and clergy during childhood. The anachronism, which is handed down from generation to generation, is remarkably pervasive among deeply religious people, despite numerous advances in science that have occurred in the past one hundred years. Deep religiosity is quite eye-catching and conspicuous among Catholic nations, like the Philippines, where at least 86% of the population, rich and poor alike, is Catholic. A similar deep devotion to Catholicism is also wide-ranging among people living in predominantly Catholic nations in South and Central America—people who were also indoctrinated (or massacred if persisting as unbelievers) – by the Spanish colonizers. In Chapter 10, I explore the possibility that epigenetic mechanisms, together with quantum mechanics, may play a role in the activation and mobilization of specific neurotransmitters in the brain during the process of indoctrination.

This book presents the scientific aspects of homosexuality. It is so appalling that, to this day, this behavior is considered a sin and even punishable by death in some major religions. Thanks to modern brain imaging, neurochemistry, endocrinology, and science of epigenetics, we now know that homosexuality has a neurobiological basis and should be treated with respect and understanding, not with ridicule and antagonism. However, a great deal of reluctance and reservation remains among some homosexuals to come out of the closet and reveal themselves openly.

In Chapter 6, I discuss the myths and facts about out-of-body (OBE) and near-death (NDE) experiences. Clearly, these phenomena, along with hallucinations and various cerebral illusory experiences, have neuroanatomical, neurochemical, and neurophysiological bases. Here, the parietal lobe is particularly relevant. This part of the brain, which is located posterior to the frontal lobe and anterior to the occipital lobe, plays a role in navigating and processing the visual and spatial orientation of the physical body. It is the somesthetic center that interprets all kinds of sensory stimuli from all parts of the body. Special attention is given to the angular and supramarginal gyri, which are parts of the parietal lobe located in the parietotemporal junction that are implicated in OBE and NDE.

Buckle up!!! Truth seekers and freethinkers will surely be intrigued and excited by the informative and scientifically factual revelations discussed in this book. Unfortunately, however, believers and religious people may react differently. They may become agitated, offended, and annoyed because most of the things I bring up in this book contradict the beliefs they acquired during childhood—that time in their lives when their limbic systems were susceptible and gullible to all types of teaching. This was particularly the case for their education in religion, where faith, along with fear of going to hell, was cultivated and nurtured through prayers recited over and over again.

The comments and opinions expressed in this book, along with much of the scientific information obtained from the numerous references listed in the bibliography, are based on my associations, over several decades, with various friends, classmates, patients, and paramedical and medical colleagues (from several institutions and different parts of the world) who have various religious beliefs and ideologies. During these many years, my close and friendly interactions with them have enabled me to analyze and understand their various personalities and religious practices. The voluminous literature on archeology, on astronomy, on ancient Sumerian, Egyptian, Mayan, Indian, and Chinese civilizations, on neurological science, and on genetics has been awe-inspiring and eye-opening. My readings provided me with the impetus to expose the hypocrisies, contradictions, paradoxes, and ironies associated with the practice of religion, all of which the devout believers fail or refuse to reconcile.

To those believers who happen to read this book, please try to be percipient. Open your other eye. May your brain synapses expand, form new neural connections, and broaden and understand the world we all live in. To laypersons who might one day become interested in reading this book, I apologize for the use of many medical and neurological terminologies, most of which have Greek and Latin roots. Many topics are covered that readers with backgrounds and expertise in neuroscience (neurologists, psychiatrists, and psychologists) may find familiar and easy to grasp, particularly topics pertaining to neuroanatomy, neurophysiology, neuropathology, and neurochemistry. I have repeated some remarks a few times during the course of presenting certain topics, but this was done on purpose to stress a point.

CHAPTER 1

The History Of Sin

"Everything that used to be a sin is now a disease." – **Bill Maher, American TV personality**

"Adam was but human—this explains it all. He did not want the apple for the apple's sake, he wanted it only because it was forbidden. The mistake was not forbidding the serpent; then he would have eaten the serpent." – **Mark Twain (1835-1910) – American writer, humorist, publisher, and lecturer**

"Homosexuality is unnatural…It says in this book, when snakes talk, people come back from the dead, a guy walks on water, and a virgin has a baby!!!" – **fb.com/WFLAtheism**

"A man's ethical behavior should be based effectually on sympathy, education, and social ties; no religious basis is necessary. Man would indeed be in a poor way if he had to be restrained by fear of punishment and hope of reward after death." – **Albert Einstein (1879-1955) – German-born theoretical physicist and developer of the theory of relativity**

"The man and woman on death row have some combination of bad genes, bad parents, bad environments, and bad ideas (and the innocent, of course, have supremely bad luck). Which of these quantities, exactly, were they responsible for? No human being is responsible for his genes or his upbringing, yet we have every reason to believe that these factors determine his character. Our system of justice should reflect an understanding that any of us could have been dealt a very different hand in life. In fact, it seems immoral not to recognize just how much luck is involved in morality itself." – **Sam Harris – neuroscientist, philosopher, and author of "The End of Faith" and "Free Will"**

Astronomers estimated that the Big Bang occurred between 12 and 14 billion years ago. "Shortly" thereafter, the Earth was born, and it is now approximately 4.5 billion years old. The Earth was extremely hot and molten during the early years of its formation, and it was quite likely that no living microorganisms or macro-organisms existed during that time. How life began during the subsequent process of development is anybody's guess. However, according to the Bible and the believers, the universe (which consists of trillions of galaxies, each containing billions of stars and billions of planets) was created by God 6000 years ago—in just 6 days!!! He apparently got tired and rested on the seventh day. Our galaxy, the Milky Way, is 100,000 light years across, and it will take 200,000 years for a spaceship to cross it at the speed of light—186,000 miles per second. It is clear that religion, as an institution based on blind faith and belief systems, and science—the systematic study of the structure and nature of the physical and natural world through experimentation and verification of laboratory data—are several light years apart and run parallel to each other, with an uncertain chance of converging.

Man's presumed ancestor apes are placed at an astonishing 25,000,000 years ago. The hominids were discovered in East Africa 14,000,000 ago. In some parts of Africa, the first ape-men (Neanderthals; h*omo neanderthalensis*) appeared 11,000,000 million years later. About 300,000 years ago, the oldest fossils of *Homo sapiens* ("thinking man") were discovered by anthropologists. *Homo sapiens* gathered food and ate animal meat, and they responded and adapted to climate and environmental challenges.

The Sumerian version of creation, occurring 4500 years ago, is quite intriguing and worthy of consideration regarding who really created humans. Sumerian clay tablets reveal that an advanced civilization was created in the land of Sumer (now modern-day Iraq), or "land of the kings." It was the first literate civilization of ancient Mesopotamia. Its people were created by gods who came down from heaven and created humans in their image in the Garden of Eden ("garden of the gods"), a place mentioned in the epic of Gilgamesh and located between the Tigris and Euphrates rivers. These gods were called the Anunnaki. The civilization they built had advanced and complex knowledge of science, mathematics, and astronomy. The humans they created lived in different cities and had organized religion and government. These gods liked to drink beer, and had prolific sex with the women of Sumeria. Each city was ruled by a powerful god.

How did an institution called religion originate? Did it exist prior to the invention of writing, which dates back to 3200 BC? If there was religion prior to that period, how was it practiced, and how did the idea of "God" originate or evolve? Polytheism, a belief in many gods, was thought to have originated with Hinduism about 2500 BC. It was also the religion of many ancient cultures, including those of Assyria, Babylonia, Egypt, Greece, and Rome. According to William Edelen (a contributor in the book titled *The Book Your Church Doesn't Want You To Read*), that famous remark, "That's where the truth is, for it was Jesus who said, I am the way, the truth and the light," is exactly the same remark Zoroaster, Buddha, and Lao Tzu of Taoism uttered. A great majority of the mythological beliefs about Christ originated from Mithraism, Zoroastrianism, Egyptian and Babylonian religions, and the Greek Mystery religions, all of which predated Christianity by several hundred to 2000 years. Around the third millennium BC, the Sumerians developed their concept of religion, but it was more akin to the concept of spirituality rather than the idea of modern religion. They believed that the universe came into existence through a series of cosmic births. In the beginning was Nammu, the primeval waters who gave birth to Ki or the Earth and An, the sky. They mated and produced a son named Enlil, who claimed Earth as his domain after separating it from heaven, and became the most dominant god. Humans were believed to have been created by Enki, the half-brother of

Enlil. Several Sumerian gods and goddesses existed, but the most well-known were An, Ki, Enlil, and Enki, who represented the personifications of the elements and natural forces. The major goddesses included Ninhursag, the goddess of fertility and the Earth, and Inanna, the goddess of sex, beauty, and warfare, who descended to the Underworld during the Akkadian Empire.

An important point to remember is that any discussion about the origin of religion entails several beliefs, ideas, thoughts, and experiences of several populations on the planet Earth, not only those of its Middle Eastern inhabitants. Immanuel Kant (1724-1804), a German philosopher and Central Enlightenment thinker, remarked, "Religious beliefs are unprovable. Religion is the product of limited empirical reasons. People are not religious due to their power of reason or their cognitive minds. On the contrary, religion is an act of the moral will. People will themselves to believe in religion—it is not the product of reason." Max Muller (1823-1900), a German-born philologist and orientalist, had a view different from Kant's. He held to the nature-worship theory, closely tied to animism. According to that theory, religion developed as primitive people observed nature, the sun, moon, wind, and rain. Their observations led to the personification of all forces of nature. This personification led to worship among the primitive people as cultures grew. Back in the pre-colonial period of the Philippines, animism was widely practiced. Ancient inhabitants believed that gods and spirits guarded rivers, forests, and mountains. Animism is the belief in spiritual beings and that the world is inhabited by spirits and supernatural entities, both good and bad. Animism was soon replaced by the Christian religion, forcibly shoved down the throats of Filipinos by the Spaniards, led by Ferdinand Magellan (a Portuguese explorer who sailed under Spanish flag) with his army of soldiers and missionaries—with Bible in one hand and sword in the other—in 1521.

The night-and-day difference in the interpretation of sin by believers and nonreligious members of the scientific community is astonishing, but understandable. The concept of sin upheld by believers totally disregards the scientific basis of human behavior, not to mention the millions of years of ape-man history that predated the Bible's version of the creation of the universe. Within the Christian teachings and traditions, seven deadly sins are included on the standard list. These are pride, greed, wrath, envy, lust, gluttony, and sloth. Acquiring wealth is part of capitalism, while wealth distribution is part of socialism, and yet the latter is an ideology that is not acceptable to people living in the free world. Regardless, all these are natural reflections of the innate makeup of the limbic system and are part of the id and ego constructs of the psychosexual development of human beings. In recent years, the Catholic Church has added a new list of sins—genetic engineering, obscene wealth, substance abuse, termination of pregnancy, pedophilia, social injustice, racism, and polluting—and these acts are exactly what Americans do (and are guilty of) every day. In regards to genetic engineering, Prince Charles, now the King of Britain, once said, "Genetic engineering takes mankind into realms that belong to God and God alone." This is a clear example of anachronism and adherence to fixed and stereotyped religious practices.

Adding pedophilia to seven deadly sins is quite appropriate and poignant. It is quite ironic that the clergy members who are supposed to be the messengers or so-called middlemen of God are the ones who often commit these despicable acts. Some of these cases were buried under the rug by fellow clerics and high members of the church hierarchy. Wrongful actions against individuals within society driven by racial prejudices remain endemic, especially in multicultural societies like the United States. Stratification of the societal structure, based on wealth and political affiliations, enhances the separation between the affluent and the poor, and between the powerful and the less influential. Family and social factors, such as physical and sexual abuse, parental neglect, peer pressure, and financial stress, put individuals at further risk for substance abuse, isolation, depression, and suicide. Environmental pollution is an inevitable consequence of progress in science and technology, but the Church's claim that it is a sin is inappropriate and narrow-minded. In all these situations, how can one define which are sinful acts, and who gets the blame—the offenders, nature, or science?

Some people say that religion, science, and politics should not be mixed. On the contrary, this is exactly what is happening in all forms of government in this world. One cannot be separated from the others, as they seem to be mutually dependent on each other. In the U.S., God is an integral part of the constitution and patriotic songs, and oaths are sworn on the Bible in the courts of law. Islamic nations are governed by powerful clerics. Strong religious influences in the Philippine government are shown by the criminalization of abortion, not to mention the prohibition of divorce in this predominantly Catholic nation. However, this mixing of religion, science and politics has always been the source of hostilities and divisions in this world. The issue of abortion and the decision to terminate pregnancy, although highly politicized, should be an individual's prerogative. The position of women and their advocates, in my opinion, should be respected; however, at the same time, terminating the life of the unborn should have some accountability. If religious advocates truly believe that such a thing as the afterlife exists, they should pray and ask their god to impose a penalty on those who terminate the lives of the unborn. It is not religious advocates' business to tell pregnant women what to do with their body.

The first description of sin dates back to the time when Adam yielded to temptation and ate the forbidden fruit that represented God's authority. By eating from the tree, he rejected God's authority. Sin was further "expanded" when Moses received the Ten Commandments from God in 1440 BCE, but other biblical scholars have no general agreement as to the exact date of Moses's encounter with God (Note: there were no witnesses when Moses received the commandments (much like Joseph Smith and the Mormons) and the people waiting for him below the mountain believed everything he told them). The redundancies in the commandments were noteworthy. This was pointed out by the late George Carlin, a brilliant stand-up comedian who grew up as an Irish Catholic in Manhattan, New York. Carlin remarked, "About five thousand years ago, a bunch of religious and political hustlers got together to figure out how they could control people and keep them in line. They knew people were basically stupid and would believe anything they were told, so these guys announced that God—God personally—had given one of them a list of Ten Commandments that he wanted to follow. They claimed the whole thing took place on a mountaintop when no one else was around." According to Carlin, the commandments should be scaled down to two—"Be honest, faithful, and loyal," and "Thou shalt not kill." He added another commandment: "Thou shalt keep thy religion to thyself." Realistically, it makes a lot of sense to scale down the commandments to two. The following commandments are all about loyalty and honesty and being faithful: "I am the Lord thy God, thou shalt not have strange Gods before me, Thou shalt not take the name of the Lord thy God in vain, Thou shalt keep holy the Sabbath, Honor thy father and mother, Thou shalt not steal, Thou shalt not bear false witness against thy neighbor, Thou shalt not commit adultery, Thou shalt not covet thy neighbor's wife, and Thou shalt not covet thy neighbor's goods".

What is quite appalling is that, despite all these commandments, we see that dishonesty, unfaithfulness, infidelity, greed, and treachery have persisted for thousands of years after they were revealed to Moses. They have always been part of life in human society. Killings in the name of religion and political ideology have remained endemic in this world for millennia. To put it in a spiritual way, sin has been on this planet from the time it was formed billions of years ago and is here to stay. Why is this so? The answer lies in the biophysical nature of sin. It is part of human behavior that is nurtured during early childhood development, molded and stored in the limbic lobe of the brain, and modulated by environmental factors.

The aforementioned sinful acts, including the infamous sexual immoralities committed by the people of two biblical and notoriously sinful cities of Sodom and Gomorrah and in the historical Nineveh, have been the basis to condemn sexual offenders as mortal sinners. Realistically, are not we all "guilty" of these "sinful" acts? Or do we all harbor various degrees of natural, but aberrant, neural connections and "rogue" neurotransmitters in our brain? Since the god of the Old Testament killed thousands and thousands of people (people he presumably created) by that great flood he himself created, did he himself commit sin? Obviously, nobody would dare ask that question because God is almighty and powerful, and he can always tell his people, "Do as I say, not do as I do." Did Cain, the firstborn son of Adam and Eve, go to hell for killing his younger brother Abel? According to the Abrahamic religion, Cain killed his brother out of jealousy and anger when God favored Abel's offering of crops over his. Why would God do an act that would lead one person to become jealous and kill another person? I thought God was fair, understanding, and just. By the way, why is it that God was visible during that time, but has not been seen interacting with humans during these modern times or during the times of war, famine, and natural disasters? What about those "religious" politicians who are involved rampantly in graft and corruption in the governments they serve. Where will their souls go? Will confession and a trip to the Vatican and Holy Shrine absolve them of their misdeeds?

Another controversial and polemical aspect of sin is how various religions view the Holy Trinity, a biblical and monotheistic doctrine, as a believable entity. The doctrine states that there are three persons, Father, Son, and Holy Spirit, in one God, and all of them are equal and simultaneously God. Robert A. Heinlein (1907-1988), science fiction writer and aeronautical engineer, remarked, "Anyone who can worship a trinity and insist that his religion is monotheism can believe anything." Very true. It is indeed difficult to mathematically imagine that one equals three, and three are one. For lack of a better reason, believers call it the "mystery of faith"—the three words always uttered by priests during mass. However, denial of the concept of the trinity is a sin, according to the Christian religion, because its denial is equivalent to non-belief in God and therefore punishable by eternal condemnation. If this is the case, will Jews, Mormons, Jehovah's Witnesses, Christian Scientists, Armstrongites, Christadelphians, Oneness Pentecostals, Unification Church members, Unity School of Christians, and Scientologists all go to hell? Robert Ingersoll (1833-1899), author of *The Foundations of Faith*, remarked, "According to the celestial multiplication table, once one is three, and three times one is one, and according to heavenly subtraction, if we take two from three, three are left. The addition is equally peculiar, if we add two to one we have but one. Each one is equal to himself and the other two. Nothing ever was, nothing ever can be more perfectly idiotic and absurd than the dogma of the Trinity."

Neuroanatomy And Neurochemistry Of Behavior

Drugs And Neurological Disorders That Alter Behavior

Religious Indoctrination Is A Wrongful Process Of Education

Hyperreligiosity Is A Form Of Obsessive-Compulsive Behavior. It Can Alter Brain Function And Anatomy

"One cubic millimeter of cerebral cortex contains roughly 50,000 neurons, each of which establishes approximately 6,000 synapses with neighboring cells. These 300 million interconnections are highly specific: Neurons innervate some target cells but avoid others. This complexity is further amplified by the fact that neurons come in many kinds. For example, some neurons make excitatory connections while others establish inhibitory ones. It is thought that there are well over 100 types of neurons that differ in shape, neurochemistry, and function. In action, each neuron integrates the signals from hundreds or thousands of synaptic signals, and this history determines whether it will send an electrical signal to its target cells." – **Harvard University https://rc.fas.harvard.edu/case-studies/connections-in-the-brain**

"Recent brain scans have shed light on how the brain simulates the future. These simulations are done mainly in the dorsolateral prefrontal cortex, the CEO of the brain, using memories of the past. On the one hand, simulations of the future may produce outcomes that are desirable and pleasurable, in which case the pleasure centers of the brain light up (in the nucleus accumbens and the hypothalamus). On the other hand, these outcomes may also have a downside to them, so the orbitofrontal cortex kicks in to warn us of possible dangers. There is a struggle, then, between the parts of the brain concerning the future, which may have desirable and undesirable outcomes. Ultimately, it is the dorsolateral prefrontal cortex that mediates between these and makes the final decisions. (some neurologists have pointed out that this struggle resembles, in

a crude way, the dynamics between Freud's ego, id, and superego.)" – **Michio Kaku, from *The Future of the Mind: The Scientific Quest to Understand. Enhance, and Empower the Mind***

"God made you in his image, really? Then why aren't you invisible?" – **atheist saying (www. geckoandfly.com)**

"The purpose of religion is not building grand temples but cultivating positive human qualities like tolerance, generosity, and love." – **Dalai Lama, Tibetan Buddhist spiritual teacher**

Common manifestations of cardiovascular and pulmonary disorders include shortness of breath, wheezing, cough, pallor, chest pain, palpitations, light-headedness, dizziness, edema, and fainting spells. Liver disorders may present with jaundice, abdominal pain, itching, change in the color of stools and urine, nausea and vomiting, body malaise, easy bruising, and decreased appetite. Manifestations of kidney disease usually include urinary frequency, bloody or foamy urine, body malaise, back or flank pain when associated with renal stones, persistent puffiness in the eyes, and edema in the legs. Common symptoms of gastrointestinal disorders include persistent diarrhea, constipation, vomiting, bloating, abdominal pain, stomach or rectal bleeding, and loss of weight, especially when associated with malignancy.

Tumors, vasculitis, infection, neurodegenerative disorders, and circulatory failure can affect the central nervous system and are manifested by various sensory and motor disturbances, such as loss of feeling and focal muscle weakness, together with seizures, headache, visual loss, speech impairment, loss of consciousness, and changes in behavior and mental function. These conditions, which disrupt the surrounding anatomical structures, are easily demonstrable by various imaging methods, such as cerebral angiograms, magnetic resonance imaging, and computerized axial tomography. However, schizophrenia, affective disorders, anxiety, and obsessive-compulsive disorders are usually diagnosed clinically because conventional imaging studies in these conditions do not show gross abnormalities. Likewise, impulsive and restrained behaviors, temperamental and stable personalities, selfishness and generosity, superiority and inferiority complexes, paranoid and trusting personalities, understanding and ignorance, bravery and cowardice, benevolence and harshness, compassion and indifference, cruelty and kindness, religious hatred and affection, rational and irrational behaviors, and racial hatred and acceptance, are contrasting traits among thinking modern humans that cannot be demonstrated by conventional radiological techniques. How can these traits be explained?

The answers lie in the various neurotransmitters and the differences in the neural interconnections in the brain, particularly in the limbic lobe. The biochemical activities in this region of the brain can be measured by functional magnetic resonance imaging (fMRI) and positron emission tomography (PET) scans. The fMRI measures brain activity by detecting changes associated with blood flow during neuronal activation, while the PET scan is a nuclear medicine technique that measures biochemical metabolic activity of the cells. The latter uses a radioactive tracer to demonstrate both normal and abnormal metabolic activity. The application of these methods has provided clinicians with valuable information about the pathophysiology and biology of various neuropsychiatric disorders, such as schizophrenia, bipolar disorder, depression, OCD, attention deficit hyperactivity disorder, and dementia. These methods also have a role in the objective assessment of therapeutic interventions and responses to therapy.

The limbic system is an arc-shaped and complex set of brain structures located on the medial and inner aspects of the cerebral hemispheres (Figure 1). The integral components of the limbic system are the cingulate gyrus, hippocampal formation, parts of the basal ganglia, amygdala, septal area, mammillary bodies, and anterior thalamic nuclei. The whole system is the seat of learning, memory, and emotion, and is tightly connected to the prefrontal cortex. It is affected in various neuropsychiatric disorders, such as schizophrenia, dementia, movement disorders, encephalitis, some forms of epilepsy, anxiety, obsessive-compulsive behavior, posttraumatic stress, posttraumatic encephalopathy, and autism. Together with the autonomic nervous system, the limbic system regulates cardiac rate, blood pressure, breathing, learning, stress, hormonal levels, and mood. One particularly interesting part of the limbic lobe is the amygdala, a cluster of neurons with an almond-like shape located in the medial temporal lobe and anterior to the hippocampus. It is also a paired structure, similar to the hippocampus. It mediates many aspects of emotion, anxiety, sexual drive, and memory. In the past, the amygdala was considered to be primarily involved in fear and other emotions related to unpleasant feelings. An exceptional behavioral disorder, known as Kluver-Bucy syndrome, affects the limbic lobe, particularly the anterior part of the temporal lobe and amygdala. This syndrome is characterized by inappropriate sexual behaviors, mouthing of objects, inability to visually recognize objects, compulsive eating, docility, seizures, memory loss, dementia, and a loss of normal fear. The condition can occur following head injury and during the course of herpes simplex encephalitis. Risk factors include Alzheimer's disease and cerebrovascular disorders.

The limbic system, as a whole, plays a key role in indoctrination processes, particular in the institution called religion, generally defined as a "quest for the value of ideal life recognition, on the part of human beings, of an almighty and controlling supernatural deity who is entitled to obedience, reverence, praise, and worship." This indoctrination process—which consists of amalgamating belief in a supernatural deity with fear of going to hell when this belief is ignored—when initiated during childhood creates permanent and almost irreversible changes in the neural circuitry of the limbic system. The information is, unfortunately, retained for life and becomes part of the instinctive mantle in the mind of the indoctrinated person. The process is solidified in subsequent years as the child grows up, especially when living in a very religious family and society. The fear of going to hell when committing perceived transgressions can cause emotional anguish, guilt, and anxiety. The vicious cycle of this process is equivalent to the kindling effect that occurs during the induction of epileptic foci in the brain. From the neurochemical standpoint, this "forced" architectural structuring of the limbic system is mediated by dopamine neurotransmitters, which act on the neural circuitry where fear conditioning has developed during the process of indoctrination. This circuitry is located in the amygdala, medial prefrontal cortex, and nucleus accumbens, along with the mesolimbic system (the midbrain, the segment of the brainstem above the pons).

> *"The majority of children born into this world tend to inherit the beliefs of their parents, and that to me is one of the most regrettable facts of them all. Let children learn about different faiths, and let them notice their incompatibility, and let them draw their own conclusions about the consequences of that incompatibility. As for whether they are "valid," let them make up their own minds when they are old enough to do so."* – **Richard Dawkins, author of *God Delusion***

Believers vehemently refuse to admit that they are victims of religious indoctrination. Recently, one classmate expressed his strong disagreement over my assertion that religious indoctrination is a wrongful process of education. He and all members of his family are devout practitioners of Catholicism. Socially and spiritually, everybody will agree that this trait is admirable and respectable, but scientifically, they exemplify the long-lasting and permanent effects of the process of indoctrination, especially when initiated during childhood. When I asked that particular classmate what religion he and his family could have adopted and practiced had they been born and grown up in Afghanistan, Indonesia, or the Himalayas, and never traveled to Western countries or to Catholic nations, he remained mum. He later sent a one-sentence letter stating that he would continue to pray for me. The implication was that I am a sinner for being a nonbeliever, but his prayer will save me from going to hell.

Recent advances in science have enabled us to understand the various human behaviors that include emotion and cognition, but some of us overlook the fact that the human body is 100% chemicals; therefore, all its physiologic functions are mediated by specialized chemical substances known as neurotransmitters—all of which are fortuitous byproducts that formed from the hot primordial soup following the "Big Bang." Several neurotransmitters are found in the brain and are either excitatory or inhibitory. The major ones are gamma aminobutyric acid, glycine, glutamate, acetylcholine, dopamine, serotonin, norepinephrine, and endorphins. The best-known neurotransmitter is acetylcholine, an ester of acetic acid and choline. It was the first neurotransmitter identified in the science of medicine; it was discovered by Henry Dale of London, England in 1914, and later confirmed by Otto Loewi of Frankfurt, Germany. Both were awarded the Nobel Prize in Medicine and Physiology in 1936. Acetylcholine is ubiquitous and is present in the peripheral and central nervous systems. It acts on the smooth muscles of the gastrointestinal tract (via the vagus and sacral nerves) and skeletal muscles (via the peripheral nerves and motor neurons) to promote contraction, and is metabolized by the enzyme acetylcholinesterase following its release from the neuromuscular junctions of the muscles. Together with the sympathetic nerves, acetylcholine released from the vagus nerves controls cardiac muscle contraction. Inhibition of the release of acetylcholine in the presynaptic segment of the neuromuscular junction, as occurs in botulism, results in paralysis, whereas blockage of its action at the postsynaptic terminals, as in myasthenia gravis, results in muscle weakness or even paralysis. Excess activity of this neurotransmitter, resulting from toxins and mushroom poisoning, is manifested by increased muscle activity (abdominal cramps), bradycardia, bronchoconstriction, increased glandular secretions, vomiting, headache, and confusion.

Acetylcholine also has a well-known presence in the brain, particularly in the nucleus basalis of the basal forebrain inferior to the anterior commissure and globus pallidus and in the pedunculopontine nucleus. These nuclei have extensive connections to various parts of the cerebral cortex and hippocampus, mediated by their rich acetylcholine content, and they control cognitive and memory function, attention, movement, and posture. These brain regions are particularly vulnerable to aging, Alzheimer's disease, and Parkinson's disease—conditions that are characterized by memory and cognitive dysfunction. The rationale behind the use of pharmacologic agents as treatment is based on their ability to augment the action of acetylcholine, the neurotransmitter that encodes and enhances memory. The nuclei that synthesize acetylcholine, dopamine, serotonin, and norepinephrine are listed in Table 1. These neurotransmitters are transported via neural projections to several centers in the cerebrum, cerebellum, and spinal cord.

Another well-known neurotransmitter is dopamine, which originates in the substantia nigra (SN) of the midbrain and ventral tegmental area (VTA) and has an important role in modulating motor movements and reward-directed behavior. Certain dopamine neurons in the VTA are activated by aversive events and promote phasic increases in the medial prefrontal cortex and nucleus accumbens. The SN connects with nuclei of the nigrostriatal pathway, which is critically involved in motor and mental deficits in Parkinsonism, Huntington's disease, Tourette's syndrome, schizophrenia, attention deficit disorder, and obsessive compulsive disorder. It became the focus of attention among neuroscientists, led by the late Greek scientist, Dr. George Cotzias (1918-1977), during the early 1960s, when a deficiency of dopamine stemming from degeneration of dopaminergic neurons in the substantia nigra of the midbrain was found to result in Parkinsonism, a condition characterized by tremor, stiffness, rigidity, paucity of movements, low voice volume, slow gait, and various gastrointestinal symptoms. Other types of Parkinsonism are characterized by dementia, delirium, and depression (Lewy Body Disease) or by motor neuron disease (Parkinsonism-Dementia-ALS complex). In subsequent years, an involvement of dopamine was found in memory, pleasure, motivation, cognition, attention, sleep, arousal, mood, and learning. Dopamine is part of the reward system that is activated when a person is addicted to certain foods that trigger the release of large amounts of dopamine. Dopamine is also released by the hypothalamus and, along with norepinephrine, is involved in the "fight-or-flight" syndrome in response to stressful or dangerous situations. Other conditions related to dopamine are restless leg syndrome—a dopamine-dependent disorder characterized by uncontrollable urge to move—and attention deficit hyperactivity disorder. Interestingly, some people suffering from Parkinsonism and receiving levodopa therapy may develop compulsive gambling behavior associated with hypersexuality months after initiation of therapy. Hyperdopaminergic activity and neurotransmitter imbalances in the limbic lobe are believed to be the underlying causes. According to Christian teachings, God hates greed, and since gambling is a form of greed, it is considered a sin. Therefore, if a person develops compulsive gambling resulting from abnormal dopamine levels in the brain, is that person committing a sin?

Any discussion about greed is incomplete without mentioning the gold and wealth, worth billions, amassed by former dictator of the Philippines who ruled the country during the late 1970s and early 1980s. He has multiple bank accounts worth billions of dollars all over the world, enough to pay the country's massive debt. He used his wealth to exert plutocratic influence to have his own men elected in the government so he could stay in power. Similar to compulsive gambling and drug addiction, greed is also dopaminergically mediated and is considered a learned form of pleasure-seeking reward. Greed is fueled by dopamine released into the nucleus accumbens (in synchrony with various nuclei in the limbic system), the pleasure center of the brain (shown in Figure 1). When it comes to money, Wall Street is the place where greed is the norm, and where some politicians acquire excessive amounts of money outside of the salary they receive from the government they run. Money is downright addicting. Greed is an age-old human behavior and is called avarice when pursued to an extreme degree.

Serotonin, a diverse monoamine neurotransmitter, is stored in and released from the median raphe nuclei, a collection of neurons positioned in the midline aspect of the brainstem and extending from the midbrain down to the pons and medulla. The nerve fibers originating from the nuclei project to the hippocampus, thalamus, hypothalamus, basal ganglia, cortex, and spinal cord. The precursor of serotonin is L-trytophan, an essential amino acid. Once released to the synaptic cleft from the presynaptic segments, serotonin is deactivated through a reuptake mechanism. Ninety percent of serotonin is primarily found in the mucosae of the gastrointestinal tract (regulation of intestinal movements), 8% in platelets (stored and released during agitation and vasoconstriction), and 1–2% in the central nervous system. Neuropsychiatrically, serotonin regulates mood, the sleep-wake cycle, body temperature, pain, social and sexual behavior, memory and learning, and appetite. Neural connections of the raphe nuclei reach almost every part of the nervous system, including the entire brain, cerebellum, and spinal cord. The psychopathology of major depression is linked to a decrease in serotonin input to the limbic system; hence, various antidepressants are serotonin reuptake inhibitors (SSRIs). Inhibition of the reuptake mechanism lengthens the duration of serotonin action. Because of the role of serotonin in social behavior, SSRIs have been used to treat impulsive aggression and violence, a condition that may be associated with decreased serotonin transmission. This association may be simplistic because other intermediary factors and chemicals come into play in the psychopathology of aggressive social behavior, including the association between violent behavior and chronic marijuana use. Moreover, various pharmacologic agents can induce aggressive and violent behavior. These include amphetamines, several antidepressant and anxiolytic agents that prolong the duration of action of serotonin and norepinephrine, triazolam (halcyon) used for insomnia, atomoxetine (strattera) for attention deficit hyperactivity disorder, and varenicline (chantix) for the treatment of nicotine addiction.

Any disease process or pharmacological treatment that can lead to imbalance and dysregulation of various neurotransmitters resulting from loss of neural networks in the limbic system can lead a person to behave differently. This situation is seen in some people suffering from Alzheimer's dementia, brain tumors, and chronic posttraumatic encephalopathy. Similar neurochemical dysfunctions may explain the behavior of some people with borderline personality disorder associated with self-mutilation (deliberate self-harm) and suicidal tendencies, conditions that are treated with serotonin reuptake inhibitors, such as sertraline (zoloft), fluoxetine (prozac), paroxetine (paxil), citalopram (celexa), and escitalopram (lexapro),

Serotonin plays an important role in other neurological conditions, including migraine headache. This common condition can be treated with triptans, a group of synthetic serotonin receptor agonists with high affinity for the 5-hydroxytriptamine receptors that are present in the smooth muscles of the blood vessels that dilate during an acute migraine attack. However, when combined with antidepressant drugs that increase or prolonged the action of serotonin, a condition known as hyperserotonin syndrome, can potentially occur. It is characterized by tremor, agitation, tachycardia, tachypnea, sweating, confusion, and delirium. It is treatable by discontinuing or reducing the dosage of the antidepressant drug or by using another abortive drug for migraine. Severe symptoms require hospitalization.

Biochemically, after serotonin is produced from L-trytophan through the process of hydroxylation and decarboxylation, it is then converted to melatonin through the process of acetylation and methylation. This process takes place within the pineal gland, a structure located in the center of the brain. The pineal gland regulates the circadian rhythm by secreting melatonin during the dark hours of the day. Low serotonin activity has been implicated in insomnia and depression. However, the physiology of sleep is a complex process that involves more than just the serotonin–melatonin pathway and may require other neurotransmitters, especially dopamine, as dopamine deficiency causes sleep disturbance as a Parkinsonism symptom.

Norepinephrine, a largely excitatory neurotransmitter, is synthesized in the nucleus of locus coeruleus (Latin, meaning "blue spot"), a brain structure located in the pons (Latin, meaning "bridge"), which is caudal to the midbrain, rostral to the medulla, and ventral to the cerebellum. The neural connections of locus coeruleus include the spinal cord, cerebellum, lateral hypothalamus, cingulate gyrus, amygdala, and medial prefrontal cortex. Norepinephrine is involved in responses to stress and panic, and it induces insomnia, anxiety, and agitation during drug withdrawal. It plays a major role in arousal and the sleep-wake cycle, emotions, attention, and memory. The locus coeruleus, together with the substantia nigra, degenerate in Parkinson's disease (PD), thereby explaining the various neuropsychiatric symptoms associated with this disease and with Lewy Body Dementia (LBD). Peripherally, norepinephrine is secreted and released into the bloodstream from the adrenal medulla, where it acts as a hormone for the part of the sympathetic nervous system that regulates the cardiovascular, gastro-intestinal, hepatic, skeletal, muscle, ocular, and integumentary systems. LBD is the second most common type of dementia, after Alzheimer's disease. Pathologically, it is characterized by deposits of protein, known as Lewy bodies, in the neurons that mediate cognition, memory, and movements. Its symptoms, which consist of tremor, muscle rigidity, slow movement, and shuffling gait, may resemble those of PD. However, the presence of visual, auditory, and olfactory hallucinations and delirium distinguishes LBD from PD. Robin Williams, a talented comedian-actor, died of LBD.

An equally, if not the most fascinating behavioral disorder is OCD, which began to be recognized during the 19th century. It is a relatively common and disabling psychiatric disorder with significant morbidity and varying severity. Recent studies have shed light on the biochemical pathology of this condition. It is an anxiety-driven condition that displays as a pattern of unwanted thoughts, fears, and urges that lead the person to engage in repetitive behaviors. Examples are checking and re-checking, compulsive hand washing, counting, arranging, hoarding, a perfectionistic attitude, sexual preoccupation, self-image preoccupation, and repetitive activities. Scrupulosity (or religious OCD) is a form of OCD that drives a person to feel guilty and sinful if he or she violates a religious doctrine. Hyperreligiosity is the result of a vicious cycle of obsessions, pathological guilt, anxiety, and reinforcement that causes a person to become imprisoned in a steel cage of religion. Common to almost all hyperreligious people is their tendency to demonize and ostracize nonbelievers when their beliefs are challenged or criticized. Genetics appears to have some influence, but despite efforts to explore the genetic basis of OCD or its associated environmental factors, its pathogenesis remains unknown. Over the years, disruption in the balance between gamma aminobutyric acid and glutamate in the cingulate cortex, together with dysregulation of the glutaminergic neurons, has been implicated in the intriguing behavioral patterns in OCD. Anatomically, many investigators have hypothesized that OCD involves dysfunction in the neural loop that interconnects the orbitofrontal cortex to the cingulate gyrus, caudate nucleus, putamen, globus pallidus, and thalamus. In severe cases that are recalcitrant to therapy, neurosurgical treatment has provided support for this hypothesis. Symptomatic relief has been achieved by means of cingulotomy, anterior capsulotomy, subcaudate tractotomy, ablation of neuronal circuitry using stereotactic radiosurgery (gamma knife) and MR-guided high-intensity focused ultrasound, and deep brain stimulation of the bed nucleus of the stria terminalis. Because of the complexity of neuronal connections in the limbic system and basal ganglia, together with the ubiquitous nature of glutamate, an excitatory neurotransmitter, establishing the exact pathophysiology of OCD remains far on the horizon.

There is no smidgen of doubt that the neurotransmitters synthesized and contained in the limbic system, with its widespread connections are what determine the human personality—not the soul. This is understandable considering that animals (and even plants) are 100% chemicals and the byproducts of the endless evolutionary processes that began 4.5 billion years ago (not 6000 years ago). One would then ask this question: If everything resides in the soul or spirit, as claimed by the believers, what is the point of having the most complex organ, along with trillions of molecules of neurotransmitters and countless synapses, protected by the cranial vault in this universe?

Hyperreligiosity, as the name indicates, is an extreme form of devotion to religion and belief in God. The believer always experiences a feeling of guilt and anxiety every time an apparent transgression is committed. I recall one patient of mine who used to see me for follow up of a chronic neurological disorder affecting her peripheral nerves. Frequently, during each clinic visit, I observed her crying and looking miserable. One day, when I asked why, she told me she had committed a sin by missing a religious congregation a week prior to the visit. At other times, she would openly express deep remorse over some venial sins she had committed since her previous office visit. Each time, at the end of the clinic visit, she would give me several passages from the Bible and pictures of Jesus Christ and the Virgin Mary, in addition to sending me other religious items, such as small wooden crucifix and rosary, during religious holidays. This condition is, unmistakably, scrupulosity. In her particular situation, it interfered with her social function and activities of daily living. Unfortunately, I lost her to follow-up and did not get a chance to evaluate her further for the possibility of concurrent conditions, such as complex partial seizure and other brain disorders characterized by hyperreligiosity.

Pathological conditions associated with hyperreligiosity include temporal lobe epilepsy (now known as complex partial seizures), psychosis in bipolar disorder, hallucinogen addiction, schizophrenia, frontotemporal dementia, and anti-NMDA receptor encephalitis. People with complex partial seizures, however, may not exhibit hyperreligiosity during the interictal period, but 0.4% and 3.1% of partial epilepsy had ictal religious experiences. One other neurological disorder presenting with hyperreligiosity is Geschwind syndrome, which is characterized by seizures, hypergraphia, hyposexuality, circumstantiality, and emotional irritability. The syndrome has been seen in frontotemporal lobe degeneration. In one case reported in 2017 by a group of investigators in Spain, a 60-year-old woman presented with hyperreligiosity and personality changes and was later found to have a malignant tumor in the right prefrontal region, with inflammatory involvement of the temporal lobe. An interesting point to note is that, throughout history, epileptic patients and their experiences during the attacks have been associated with divine and supernatural connotations and demonic possession. It is so appalling to consider that numerous pathologic events, like those observed among epileptics in ancient civilizations, became the basis of belief systems and fanaticisms in some religious organizations.

Anti-NMDA Receptor Encephalitis is a rare autoimmune encephalitis characterized by complex neuropsychiatric and systemic symptoms, such as fever, headache, malaise, agitation, confusion, fluctuations in blood pressure and cardiac rate, delusions, hallucinations, hyperreligiosity, and seizures. Half of the cases are associated with tumors, most commonly ovarian teratomas. The estimated number of cases is one in 1.5 million people per year. The disease affects women of childbearing age. The pathologic mechanism involves the presence of immunoglobulin G antibodies against the NR1 subunit of the NMDA receptors in the brain. Diagnosis is achieved by detecting the presence of antibodies in the spinal fluid. It is treated with the use of immunosuppressive agents. Early surgical removal of the tumor, if present, offers good prognosis in about 80% of cases.

What does religion do to the brain? Does it induce, facilitate, promote, worsen, and exacerbate delusionary ideas and hallucinations in some people at risk for developing psychosis, those who are already psychotic, those who are deeply religious, and those with early neurodegenerative disorders? Whether a divine powerful being exists is a matter of opinion, but it is a scientific fact that religion can alter the anatomical, physiological, and chemical makeup of the brain. Dr. Andrew Newberg, professor of neuroscience at Thomas Jefferson University, indicated that "different religious practices have different effects on one's brain." In a clinical and radiological study performed by a group of investigators led by Dr. Amy D. Owen of Duke University, using high-resolution MRI on a sample of 268 older adults and correlating the findings with religious factors and structural neuroanatomy, significantly greater hippocampal atrophy was observed in participants reporting a life-changing religious experience. Significantly greater hippocampal atrophy was also observed from baseline to final assessment among born-again Protestants, Catholics, and those with no religious affiliation, compared with Protestants not identifying as born-again. The authors hypothesized that the atrophy of the hippocampus was related to stress hormones that are released during the time of stress, similar to findings in people who live a stressful life. This study contradicts the positive effects of religion in some individuals, but it reveals the complex relationship between religion and the brain.

Another constellation of symptoms stemming from rigorous and prolonged religious indoctrination processes is called "Religious Trauma Syndrome," a condition characterized by cognitive dysfunction, disturbances in affect, functional disturbances, and sociocultural difficulties. The act of leaving the controlling and authoritarian dogmatic religious community is a major factor in the genesis of symptoms. The symptoms include confusion, difficulty in decision-making, depression, sadness, suicidal thoughts, guilt feelings, loss of self-esteem, anxiety, polarity in emotion (anger and grief), seclusion, sexual problems, and loss of orderliness in activities of daily living. Recommended treatments include cognitive behavioral therapy, prolonged exposure therapy, eye movement desensitization and reprocessing, somatic therapy, faith-based therapy, and radically open dialectical behavior therapy.

Looking at all these recent scientific studies, could it be that the countless atrocities—those committed by Christians against persons who refused to accept their religion (i.e., the millions of Jews killed by Adolph Hitler, a Catholic), the thousands of Christians killed by dictators and tyrants, and the thousands of Americans killed in 9/11 bombing—would not have happened if not for religious indoctrination and fanaticism? "Religion does three things: Divides people, controls people, deludes people." – Carlespie Mary Alice McKinney, essayist and business professor.

Diagram of the limbic system

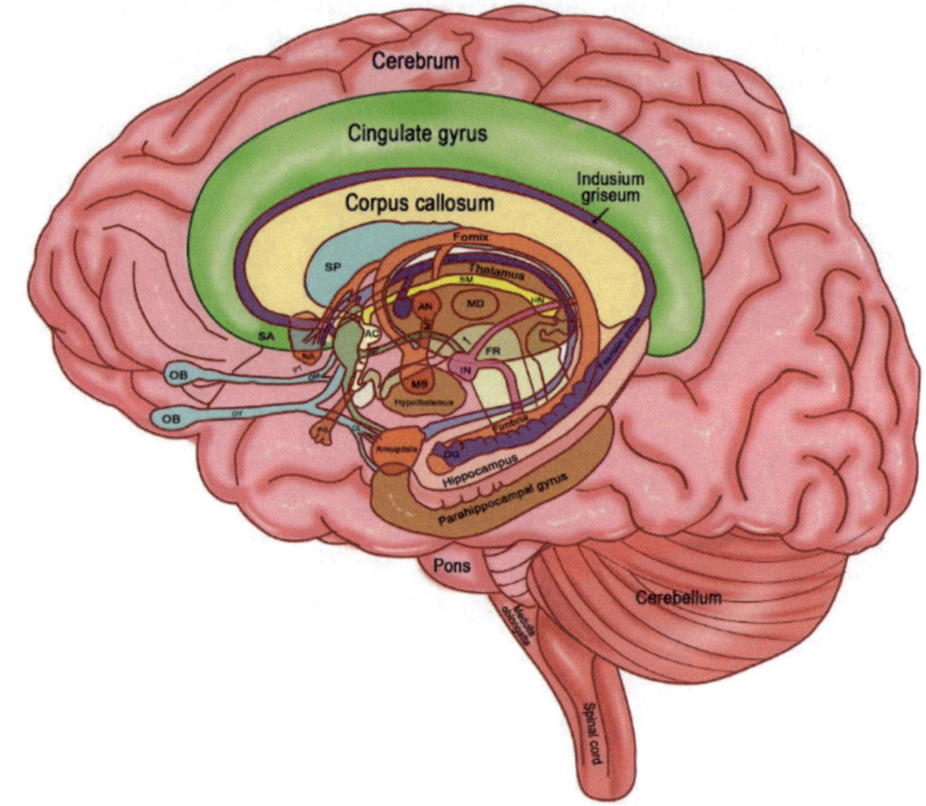

Cutout anatomy diagram of the human limbic system and some neighboring structures – Modified from the original source – John Taylor. General Science (https://web.archive.org/web/20130609090504/http://tayloredge.com/reference/Science

Abbreviations: AC – Anterior commissure, AN – Anterior nucleus of thalamus, DG – Dentate gyrus, FR –Fasciculus retroflexus, IN – Interpeduncular nucleus, LT – Lamina terminalis, MB – Mammillary body, MD – Mediodorsal thalamic nucleus, MF – Medial forebrain bundle, MT – Mammilothalamic tract, NA –Nucleus accumbens, OB – Olfactory bulbs, OC – Optic chiasm, OL – Olfactory striae lateral, OS – Olfactory striae medial, OT – olfactory tract, PG – Pituitary gland, PT – Paraterminal gyrus, SA – Subcallosal area, SM – Stria medullaris, SN – Septal nuclei, SP – Septum pellucidum, ST – Stria terminalis

TABLE 1
MAJOR NEUROTRANSMITTERS OF THE BRAIN

Origins	Projections
ACETYLCHOLINE	
1. NUCLEUS BASALIS AND MEDIAL SEPTAL NUCLEI	Neocortex Hippocampus
2. PEDUNCULOPONTINE AND LATERODORSAL TEGMENTAL NUCLEI	Brainstem Thalamus Cerebellum
DOPAMINE	
1. VENTRAL TEGMENTAL AREA OF THE MIDBRAIN	Tuberoinfundibular pituitary pathway Mesolimbic pathway Nucleus Accumbens Hypothalamus Mesocortical pathway
2. SUBSTANTIA NIGRA OF THE MIDBRAIN	Dorsal palliudum (globus pallidus) Thalamus Putamen
SEROTONIN	
MEDIAN RAPHE NUCLEI OF THE BRAINSTEM	Hippocampus Thalamus Hypothalamus Basal Ganglia Cortex Spinal cord
NOREPINEPHRINE	
LOCUS COERULEUS OF ROSTRAL PONS AND THE LATERAL FLOOR OF THE FOURTH VENTRICLE	Lateral hypothalamus Amygdala Cingulate gyrus Hippocampus Thalamus Neocortex and medial prefrontal cortex Cerebellum Spinal cord

Religious Views On Sin

Science And Crime

Medical And Legal Aspects Of Sin

Homosexuality

"There is a fundamental difference between religion, which is based on authority, [and] science which is based on observation and reason. Science will win because it works." – **Stephen Hawking (1942-2018), British theoretical physicist and cosmologist**

"Science is based on experiment, on a willingness to challenge the old dogma, on an openness to see the universe as it really is. Accordingly, science sometimes requires courage to question the conventional wisdom." – **Carl Sagan (1934-1996), American astronomer, cosmologist, and planetary scientist**

"Adversity is the first path to truth" – **Lord Byron (1788-1824), English poet and lyricist**

"Christianity has done its utmost to close the circle and declared even ***doubt*** *to be sin. One is supposed to be cast into belief without reason, by a mistake, and from then on to swim in it as in the brightest and least ambiguous of elements: even a glance towards land, even the thought that are perhaps exists for something else as well as swimming, even the slightest impulse of our amphibious nature—is sin! And notice that all this means that the foundation of belief and all reflection on its origin is likewise excluded as sinful. What is wanted are blindness and intoxication and an eternal song over the waves in which reason has drowned."* – **Friedrich Nietzsche, in "Daybreak: Thoughts on the Prejudices of Morality"**

From the beginning, the introduction of the concept of sin was likely meant to control the minds of the naturally violent humans born into a society that promotes and encourages hostility and greed, and into an environment that serves the human ego. To spiritualists and religious people, a sinful act is wrong—a transgression against divine law. To the corporealists, like neuroscientists, that act is simply a natural human behavior that reflects the biological activities of the neurons in the limbic system in response to outside stimuli. It is punishable if considered a crime, as determined by the laws of the land where the person lives, unless the person is exonerated by reason of insanity. From a religious standpoint, the punishment is eternal torture in hell. This punishment is imposed on the soul of the person who committed the sinful act. That soul is a non-organic and independent entity that supposedly controls mood and emotion—a strong and firm conviction that spiritualists and believers passionately maintain. Unfortunately, this conviction has no scientific basis, and the presumed existence of something that cannot be perceived by special senses is difficult to accept as factual.

In the past 50 years, advances in neuroscience have grown exponentially, enabling modern society to get a better understanding of human behavior and to determine if a given behavior is within or outside the standard or accepted societal way of life. We have now identified the neuronal populations in the brain, together with several neurotransmitters, that mediate and control behavior. This behavior can be changed or modulated through the use of various drugs that can either excite or inhibit the activity of the neurotransmitters that are synthesized and transported to various neural networks in the brain. Obviously, none of this information was available to ancient civilizations, but it is quite ironic and illogical that modern day society continues to propagate knowledge obtained through a belief system—a system that originated from hearsay propagated and handed down from one generation to another by a scientifically and technologically unsophisticated ancient civilization. Go figure.

Retrospectively, given the absence of science among people in the distant past, one might wonder how many of the so-called "crimes" or "sins" committed by people behaving "badly" were actually committed by persons harboring neurons with aberrant neural connections in their brains or with degenerative brain disorders, epilepsy, neoplasm, microbial infections, or hallucinogenic plant intoxications that drove them to commit the criminal or sinful act. Today, culpability and guilt in murder cases are based on wanting to commit a crime (as in a crime of passion), as opposed to urges to murder people in association with mental illnesses like paranoid schizophrenia or the aggressive and violent behaviors associated with chronic marijuana use. In disease cases, the presence of a disorder can be used in a court of law as a mitigating circumstance that lessens the degree of criminal culpability. Either way, killing another person is simply not commonplace and the person who commits such act is frequently viewed with contrasting and diverging attitudes—with condemnation by the lay public versus scientific percipience and understanding by some professionals who are aware that neural aberrancies in the limbic system can drive a person to commit crimes.

The Abrahamic religions of Judaism, Christianity, and Islam have a uniform concept of sin, which is based on the Ten Commandments revealed to Moses by God at Mount Sinai, and on the so-called original sin committed by Adam and Eve in the Garden of Eden, as revealed in the Old Testament. Depending on the degree of the sin, it is either forgivable or punishable by eternal damnation. Buddhism, the world's fourth-largest religion that originated in ancient India, has no concept of sin or of the original sin understood in some religions. According to the Buddhist principle, all human actions are subject to the universal moral code or reign of law, but not to the moral standards set forth by the god of Abrahamic religions. As a matter of fact, Buddhism has no concept of a divine creator, as defined by monotheist religions. In essence, it is a non-theistic religion. Strictly speaking, the terms "theist and atheist" should not even exist, because they presuppose the existence of a creator god. The terms came into existence when the concept of god was propagated by most major religions. According to the laws of most major religions, unbelief or denial of the existence of that supreme god is a punishable offense. Therefore, will the nontheist people like the Buddhists be punished or go to hell? Is it their fault for not believing in a supreme creator? Is it the fault of Buddhist parents who never inculcated the idea of the Abrahamic god into the limbic systems of their children?

Numerous anatomical, clinical, and imaging data implicate the entire limbic system, including the thalamus and basal ganglia, in the control of cognition and emotion. All these structures are interconnected to each other, as shown by two advanced magnetic resonance imaging techniques: diffusion tensor tractography (DTI) and resting-state functional connectivity. The latter radiological technique detects temporal correlations in the oscillations of the blood oxygenation level between brain regions while patients rest quietly on the scanner table. This technique shows the areas of heightened activity in the cingulate gyrus in patients with depression. By contrast, DTI demonstrates nerve fiber tracts that constitute the white matter. It analyses the microstructural integrity of these fiber tracts, including the axons, in traumatic brain injuries and small vessel disease. It also measures disease severity in the cognitively impaired.

Traumatic brain injury (TBI) and its long-term sequelae have been the focus of attention among various medical specialties and the legal system. The most frequent cause is closed head injury resulting from acceleration-deceleration injuries to several parts of the brain, particularly the frontal lobe. Disturbance in executive function owing to bruising of the orbitofrontal cortex is common. The effects of TBI can result from a cascade of axonal degenerations (a domino effect) along the pathways that interconnect the frontal lobe with the rest of the cerebral cortex, brainstem, and corpus callosum. The disconnections that result from TBI result in executive dysfunction similar to that seen in disorders that affect the white matter, such as multiple sclerosis, lupus erythematosus, small vessel disease related to hypertension, cerebral amyloid angiopathy or diabetes, neoplasms, surgical and radiation treatments, schizophrenia, obsessive-compulsive disorder, Tourette's syndrome, and borderline personality disorder. For example, cognitive, behavioral, and various motor abnormalities are well known to occur among boxers. The condition has various terms, such as "punch drunk," "goofy," "slug-nutty," and dementia pugilistica. TBI is the result of repeated blows to the head. It is now termed chronic traumatic encephalopathy (CTE) because, as has become clear in recent years, the condition has emerged in association with sports injuries, particularly football and soccer, and situations that cause repeated head trauma and falls, such as epileptic spells, head banging, and physical abuse.

Early manifestations of CTE include depression, irritability, polarity in emotion, temperamental outbursts, poor episodic memory, cognitive dysfunction, poor judgment, and apathy. Suicidal ideation may soon follow. Dementia, movement disorders, and signs of parkinsonism are terminal features. Associations with increased risk of violence, suicidal behavior, and earlier age of conviction and incarceration have been reported. These are compounded by family issues that include alcoholism, drug addiction, physical and sexual abuse, and genetically mediated psychiatric issues.

Macroscopic pathologic features of CTE include atrophy of the frontal and temporal cortices, medial temporal lobe, mammillary bodies, cerebellum, basal ganglia, and hypothalamus. Microscopically, pathologic findings include neurofibrillary and glial tangles, features seen in Alzheimer's disease and other tauopathies, beta amyloid deposits and plaques, and widespread TDP-43 proteinopathy. Lewy bodies (LB) are also seen in various parts of the neocortex and limbic system, particularly in the amygdala. LB are abnormal aggregates of alpha-synuclein protein found inside the neurons of patients suffering from dementia and various movement disorders.

Reports of violent behavior and murders committed by athletes, such as football players, suffering from CTE have sounded alarms and raised concerns in several sectors of society. Some of these players who became depressed ended up committing suicide after killing a family member. Some, including several boxers, died owing to complications of dementia years after they retired from playing or fighting. CTE is clearly a potential cause of criminality. Did those athletes who suffered and died from CTE and killed their loved ones commit a sin? Will they be punished in hell? Scientifically, in the true sense of the word, are they really criminals?

Scientific studies have shown abnormalities in the brains of murderers. Using positron emission tomography, one study demonstrated reduced glucose metabolism in several parts of the limbic system (prefrontal cortex, corpus callosum, thalamus, amygdala, and medial temporal lobe, along with the superior parietal gyrus and left angular gyrus) of murderers. While mental health issues, such as depression and substance abuse (and particularly chronic use of marijuana) are risk factors, they appear to make up a small percentage of the overall risk factors. Therefore, one cannot quantify the role of mental illness in the occurrence of mass murders. Regardless, the people who commit violent crimes may harbor pathologic anatomical and neurochemical substrates in their limbic system, particularly in the orbitofrontal cortex. Do these people with abnormalities in their limbic systems who commit violent crimes and mass murders go to hell? The mainstream media have always been quick to label these crimes as "pure evil," while totally ignoring the scientific aspects of the acts that led to the crimes.

Mental disabilities, insanities, and even the presence of an extra "Y" chromosome have been used by defense lawyers to lessen the criminal culpability of their clients. These issues are always complex, and they always generate controversies and confusion, especially among people who are either religious and/

or scientifically unsophisticated. When crime and science intersect, valuable information provided by the latter frequently benefits both the prosecution and the defense panel. The acquittal of a person who has committed mass murder by a court of law when the medical evidence proves that the person was suffering from paranoid schizophrenia can be quite difficult for the victims' family members to accept. Years ago, this would have been considered a sinful act, and the person who committed the heinous act would have been excommunicated or sentenced to death. The advent of sophisticated imaging studies has enabled scientists to understand why some people behave badly and why others are able to live harmoniously with their fellow humans. Criminal offenders with psychopathic clinical features, such as antisocial behavior, impaired empathy, and egotistical traits, are often vilified and ostracized, but these are the same people with lower gray matter density in the orbitofrontal cortex and anterior insula, as demonstrated by functional MRI. Should these be people be despised and sent to prison? Should the same people, although created with defects by a supreme creator, be condemned and guaranteed to go to hell according to divine rule? What about those who commit mass murders in the name of religion or political ideologies and soldiers who kill hundreds of enemy soldiers in times of war in defense of their countries?

Religion and science have always been immiscible, despite all the numerous technological advances accomplished by the latter over the last 100 years. By contrast, religion for thousands of years has always been all about mind control, miracles, apparitions, and belief in a supernatural being who must always be praised, worshipped, and feared. Religion is a remarkably stagnant and fixated institution based on a belief system that believers feel must always be fed into their minds every day of their lives or else they pay the consequences for neglecting the daily obligation. Here is a major example that has been a hotly contentious issue in the political, social, and religious world since time immemorial. This issue concerns homosexuality, defined as a sexual attraction or behavior between members of the same sex. As stated previously, this sexual orientation is a punishable offence in some religions. It was considered a form of mental disorder by the American Psychiatric Association until 1973, when advocates and activists pressured the organization to remove the denotation. Fourteen years later, homosexuality was completely removed from the Diagnostic and Statistical Manual of Mental Disorders. It is a well-documented social behavior dating back to recorded history in ancient Greece, Rome, Egypt, India, and China, and as far back in 8000 BC in Africa. European explorers had witnessed homosexual practices among the natives in America, the Pacific Islands, and Asia. In ancient times, opposition to this behavior varied among different religions, from covert to overt rejection, to condemnation, and to punishment by stoning or even burning at the stake.

Opposition to homosexuality, in general, is frequently associated with religious conservatism. To this day, homosexuality is considered sinful and shameful by most members of the Abrahamic religions. Traditional Christianity rejects such practices without any reservations whatsoever, while others, such as liberal Christianity and Reform Judaism, view homosexuality as acceptable. Hinduism has various positions on homosexuality, ranging from supportive to neutral or outright opposition. According to Buddhist ethical laws, one should not crave sensual pleasure, and monks should refrain from sexual pleasure of any kind. Moreover, same-sex relationships are not considered a religious matter to most Buddhists. The Dalai Lama of Tibet considered lesbian and gay sex or any sex outside of penis-vaginal intercourse to be a form of sexual misconduct but, interestingly, he supports human rights for all, regardless of sexual orientation. Some Buddhists in Thailand consider homosexuality to be something innate or a condition that is congenitally acquired. Numerous countries criminalize homosexuality: Afghanistan, Algeria, Antigua and Barbuda, Bangladesh, Barbados, Bhutan, Brunei, Burundi, Cameroon, Chad, Comoros, Cook Islands, Dominica, Egypt, Eritrea, Eswatini, Ethiopia, Gambia, Ghana, Grenada, Guinea, Guyana, Iran, Jamaica, Kenya, Kiribati, Kuwait, Lebanon, Liberia, Libya, Malawi, Malaysia, Maldives, Mauritania, Mauritius, Morocco, Myanmar, Namibia, Nigeria, Palestinian Territory of Gaza Strip, Oman, Pakistan, Papua New Guinea, Qatar, Saint Kitts and Nevis, Saint Lucia, Saint Vincent and The Grenadines, Samoa, Saudi Arabia, Senegal, Sierra Leone, Singapore, Solomon Islands, Somalia, South Sudan, Sri Lanka, Sudan, Syria, Tanzania, Togo, Tonga, Tunisia, Turkmenistan, Tuvalu, Uganda, Uzbekistan, Yemen, Zambia, and Zimbabwe. Japan is the sole G7 country to ban same-sex marriage. In a recent ruling, an Osaka court has deemed that a ban on same-sex marriage is constitutional.

In this modern age, it can be quite appalling to some people who have good knowledge of the scientific aspect of human sexual orientation to think that homosexuality was, and still is, considered a crime or a sin, depending on the rules of law promulgated by some organized religions. However, a global trend is now emerging to decriminalize same-sex acts, thanks to political pressure from various advocates and activists and/or a growing knowledge of the biology, anatomy, and neurochemistry of sexual behavior. Various countries now have laws against discrimination in the workplace based on sexual orientation.

In the past twenty years, knowledge of sex differences in brain structure, gray matter density, function, and chemistry has evolved dramatically, several thousand years after incessant and unrelenting religious condemnation of homosexuality by the technologically unsophisticated ancient civilization. This relatively short period of time reflects the exponential scientific advances made in the past 100 years, particularly in the field of medicine and genetics. However, a great number of religiously indoctrinated people in this world still tenaciously and blindly adhere to their belief systems—systems that hinder scientific progress.

Sexual identity and sexual orientation are basically independent components of a person's sexual behavior and may be biologically related to prenatal factors, postnatal interactions, and socialization.

Homosexuality has always been a contentious social issue, despite the increasing tendency to accept it in mainstream society. Recent studies have shown greater gray matter volume in the thalamus and precentral gyrus in heterosexual men than in homosexual men. Physiologically, the findings show that sexual orientation correlates strongly with brain centers linked to processing and integrating afferent (incoming) sensory, reward-related, and motor information. A thinner visual cortex and smaller thalamus volumes have also been found among homosexual men. An enlarged suprachiasmatic nucleus has also been found among homosexual men. This nucleus is part of the hypothalamus that receives visual input from the optic nerve to regulate the biological clock or circadian rhythm, together with regulation of autonomic functions such as digestion, heart rate, and papillary reactions to certain stresses. In addition, the anterior commissure, a fiber tract that connects the two temporal lobes, has been found to be larger in homosexual men. Physiologically, homosexual men displayed activation of the pre-optic nucleus of the hypothalamus in response to a testosterone derivative, which shows a link between sexual orientations and the hypothalamus. Endocrinologically, sexual differentiation of the human hypothalamus and its relationship to gender identity and sexual orientation have been linked to testosterone surges during the second half of pregnancy—a surge will result in a masculine brain and absence of a surge will result in a feminine brain. The role of epigenetics in homosexuality is discussed in Chapter 10.

We are now at a crossroads whereby scientific advances in understanding homosexuality have given society a choice to either continue to disapprove this type of behavior or to find ways to accept it in our society and understand the science behind it. Unfortunately, unless religion and mainstream society—setting politics aside—begin to understand and accept the scientific bases of human behavior, criminalization of certain rogue behaviors, homosexuality, and pedophilia will remain serious and controversial issues, both socially and legally. Culpability and criminal responsibility will always be on the shoulders of those who committed the "sinful" acts, and will remain so as long as religion and science remain several light years apart.

Clergy Sexual Abuse Of Minors

"A fact never went into partnership with a miracle. Truth does not need the assistance of miracle. A fact will fit every other fact in the universe, because it is the product of all other facts. A lie will fit nothing except another lie made for the express purpose of fitting it." – **Robert Ingersoll (1833-1899), American lawyer, Civil War veteran, orator**

"Honestly, just how long must our children suffer at the hands of the deviants of God?" – **A.K. Kuykendall, American writer, Albany, Georgia**

"They like to use those fancy words. They don't like to say 'raped.' They say 'misdeed,' 'inappropriate touching,' 'mistake.' That's insulting. I'm not a mistake." – **Charles L. Bailey Jr. - author, "In the Shadow of the Cross"**

The term paraphilia is derived from the Greek (para) "beside" and (-philia) "love." It is an abnormal sexual behavior or impulse characterized by intense sexual urges that may involve unusual or non-human objects and suffering or humiliation of oneself or one's partner, non-consenting persons, and children. Behaviors that are considered paraphilias include exhibitionism, fetishism, frotteurism, sexual masochism and sadism, transvestism, voyeurism, and pedophilia. The main focus in this chapter is pedophilia, a condition formerly classified as a psychiatric disorder in which an adult or older adolescent has sexual feelings directed toward prepubescent children of either or both sexes. A related disorder, known as ephebophilia, is characterized by homosexual attraction to adolescent boys.

In recent years, pedophilia and/or sexual abuse of minors by the clergy has been an enormous public concern in society. The general public view is that the condition is a crime punishable by law. To agnostics and atheists, it represents one of the contradictions and hypocrisies in the practice of religion. To some scientists and medical professionals, it is a neuropsychiatric disorder stemming from a malfunctioning limbic system, particularly an abnormal orbitofrontal cortex (Figure 2)—the part of the brain that mediates moral-knowledge acquisition and social integration. Abnormalities associated with dysfunction of this part of the brain can result in poor impulse control, sociopathy, and altered sexual behavior. The altered behavior is treated with indifference, hatred, and ostracism. This is in sharp contrast to disorders of other organs, wherein the sufferers are treated with sympathy and compassion. The sharp divide between the maladies that affect the brain and those that affect the extracranial organs is quite remarkable.

In March 2003, an article titled, "Right Orbitofrontal Tumor with Pedophilia Symptom and Constructional Apraxia Sign," was published in the Archives of Neurology, (Volume 60, 437-440). The subject was a 40-year-old man in previous good health who developed an increasing interest in child pornography. He denied previous attraction to children, but he had a preexisting interest in pornography dating back to his adolescent years. He went to great lengths to hide his activities and continued to act on sexual impulses, but he was very much aware that his behavior was unacceptable. Later, he began making sexual advances toward his prepubescent stepdaughter. Following a legal process, he was removed from his home and underwent treatment for sexual addiction, during which time he solicited sexual favors from the staff members of the rehabilitation unit and was later removed from the unit. However, he began complaining of an increasing headache the day before his prison sentencing. Subsequent neurological evaluation revealed several frontal lobe signs and a large tumor in the anterior fossa skull base that had displaced the right orbitofrontal lobe and distorted the prefrontal cortex. The tumor was a hemangiopericytoma. This rare tumor, which accounts for less than one percent of intracranial tumors, arises from blood vessels and soft tissues. It is usually benign, but it can be invasive. It generally occurs in adults 30–50 years old. Following surgical resection of the tumor, his symptoms, including urinary bladder function, improved, enabling him to return home. A year later, the headache, together with interest in child pornography, recurred. The recurrence of the symptoms correlated with tumor regrowth that required another surgery. Following the second surgery, all his symptoms again receded. No further follow-up on the patient's condition is available.

In 2016, another case of a brain tumor with compression of the orbitofrontal cortex and hypothalamus presenting with pedophilic behavior was published in the Journal of Neurology (Volume 263, 1454-1455). The tumor, located at the base of the brain, was a clivus chordoma—a slow-growing cancerous tumor derived from cells left over from embryological development of the spine and skull. The patient was a pediatrician in his 60s and had been accused of inappropriately touching his patients. He was subsequently found to have frontal lobe abnormalities, both clinically and radiologically. It was later determined that he should not be held liable by reason of insanity.

Besides brain tumors, traumatic brain injury, particularly injuries that involve the basal frontal lobe and right fronto-temporal-insular lobes, has also been reported to lead to pedophilia and hypersexuality. Pedophilic behavior has been reported 12 to 30 years following injury to the frontal lobes. These occurrences have obvious social and legal implications.

Outside of demonstrable anatomical lesions that can lead to deviant sexual behavior, scientific studies have shown various abnormalities in different parts of the brain in pedophilia. In forensic nonviolent, inpatient pedophilic subjects, these abnormalities, as demonstrated by voxel-based morphometry and volumetry, included a significant decrease in the volume of the gray matter of the right amygdala, hypothalamus, septal regions, substantia innominata, and bed nucleus of the striae terminalis, along with enlargement of the anterior temporal horn of the right lateral ventricle. Cerebral white matter deficiencies, particularly affecting the fronto-occipital fasciculus and arcuate fasciculus, have also been demonstrated using T1-weighted magnetic resonance imaging. In another study, the right temporal gyrus was identified as a possible brain area that mediates sexual arousal in pedophilic disorder by positron emission tomography and visual sexual stimuli depicting children. During presentation of the respective sexual stimuli, the thalamus, globus pallidus, and striatum—all areas in the brain involved in sexual arousal and behavior—showed significantly greater activation among pedophiles than in controls. A recent study using functional magnetic resonance imaging revealed a significant reduction in the resting functional connectivity between the right centromedial amygdala and the left dorsolateral prefrontal cortex in child sexual offenders compared to controls.

These case reports illustrate that human behavior—good and bad—is controlled by complex neuroanatomical, neurophysiological, and neurochemical interactions in the limbic system. However, to victims of clergy sex abuse, including their relatives and the general public, this behavior is unacceptable and deplorable. Regardless of the results of scientific studies, pedophilic perpetrators will always be treated with disdain and contemptuousness. Indeed, it is grossly ironic that the ecclesiastic members of the house of worship who are supposed to relay the messages of God to humanity are the same people who would commit such diabolical and abhorrent misdeeds that will leave wounds that will never heal in the victims' psychological state. Therein lies the contradiction in an institution called religion.

Given the inordinately high incidence of clergy sex abuse, along with permanent psychological injuries inflicted on the victims, I honestly and truly empathize with the victims and their relatives. Today, numerous law firms advertise their services to these victims. They have lists of priests all over the United States who have allegedly committed sex acts against minors. Because of large financial settlements, some dioceses have filed for bankruptcy—unfortunate sequelae of an act considered both a crime and a sin but at the same time an act that may be due to aberrations in the neuronal circuitry in the brain, particularly in the frontal lobes of some clerics.

The list of clergy sexual abuse of minors has been growing in recent years, owing to close media scrutiny and public awareness. This is a global crisis that has claimed thousands and thousands of victims, leaving a permanent scar on the emotional states of the victims. It has become a widely reported story in recent years, and it has resulted in a sharp decline in trust in the members of the places of worship, particularly the Catholic Church. The incidence is particularly inordinately high in predominantly Catholic nations. In the Philippines, where at least 86% of citizens are Roman Catholics, several hundred priests suspected of committing sexual misconduct with minors have been investigated by the Catholic bishops. Notably, some sexual abuses were committed against adults. One victim, a 14-year-old girl, was raped repeatedly in 1997 by a Filipino priest. One independent inquiry in France concluded that over 200,000 persons were victims of sexual abuse carried out by the clergy of the French Catholic Church between 1950 and 2020. Reports of allegations of sexual abuse have spread across several European countries, such as Germany, Netherlands, Austria, Spain, Switzerland, and Portugal. In Poland, the Polish Bishops' Conference reported 624 victims of clergy sex abuse that occurred between 1990 and 2018. In Brazil, it was reported that 10% of the country's clergy were sex offenders.

Several thousand Catholic clergy members in the United States have been accused of sexual abuse that dates back decades. In 2002, the Boston Globe reported that church officials had uncovered 130 cases of sexual abuse committed by a former priest during a three-decade period while serving in several Boston parishes. In Pennsylvania, the ProPublica database includes 76 abusers from the Archdiocese of Philadelphia, 108 abusers from the Diocese of Pittsburgh, 50 abusers from the Diocese of Allentown, 83 abusers from the Diocese of Scranton, 72 abusers from the Diocese of Harrisburg, 94 abusers from the Diocese of Erie, 21 abusers from the Diocese of Greensburg, and 35 abusers from the Diocese of Altoona-Johnstown. Clearly, these acts committed by the clergy are loathsome, but have you ever wondered how many of those clerics from yesteryears, including those who were canonized saints, were harboring rogue neurons in their limbic systems or were suffering from either benign or malignant tumors in their brains?

Cruelty in the name of religion has been well documented in world history. On March 29, 2022, the Daily Gazette of Schenectady, New York, published an article titled "Indigenous tell Pope of abuses endured at Canada School." It reported that more than 150,000 tribal children were isolated from their native culture and forced to attend residential schools run by Catholic missionaries. They were beaten and physically and sexually abused by the clergy from the 19th century until the 1970s for speaking their native languages. The pope recently apologized to the indigenous people of Canada in a recent visit in the early summer of 2022.

Questions have been raised about the strict adherence to—what some critics believe—the controversial and unfair practice of male-only priesthood in the Catholic religion. The most common explanation for this practice is that the apostles were all men. Those in the higher hierarchy of Catholic religion deny sexism 2000 years ago as the root cause, and they simply claim that women cannot perform the basic function of priesthood. Simply put, it means that women cannot be sacramental symbols of Jesus Christ—who himself might have been a male chauvinist or possibly a homosexual. In this modern era of a strong feminist movement and political correctness, this exclusionary practice is considered egotistical, selfish, and politically incorrect. The higher echelons of the Catholic hierarchy will not admit the fact that women in ancient times, and even some religions to this day, were considered second class citizens and subservient to their spouses. What if women are allowed to become priests? Would this affect the incidence of pedophilia in the Catholic religion? The strict adherence to a male-only priesthood is appalling. In 2002, an independent international organization that claimed a connection with the Roman Catholic Church organized a group called "Roman Catholic Womenpriests." It was a group of women who asserted that they were ordained as priests by

Romulo Antonio Braschi and two other unnamed bishops. The group was eventually excommunicated by the Vatican.

Realistically, the likelihood that sexual abuse of minors may be due to aberrant or abnormal circuitry in the limbic system of the offenders is something that the lay public is reluctant to accept as a valid explanation for the abhorrent and loathsome behavior by the clergies. To the traditional religious followers of faith, these acts are sinful and unacceptable and must be punished by eternal damnation and/or incarceration. Although this sentiment is understandable, modern society should be aware that clear, objective, and factual evidence supports the idea that human behavior is mediated and controlled by groups of neurons in the limbic formation of the central nervous system, as explained in the foregoing discussion. This situation creates a sharp division between the emotional and deplorable aspects of such acts against minors versus the science behind the deviant behavior.

An interesting genetic and epigenetic aspect of pedophilia is discussed in CHAPTER 9.

Orbitofrontal cortex and limbic system

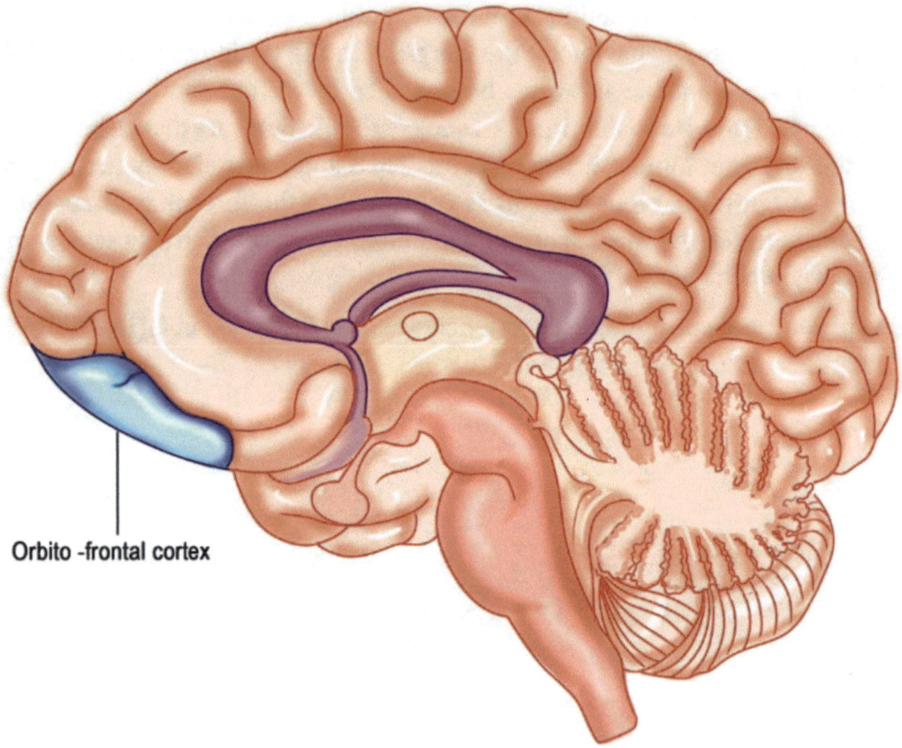

Orbitofrontal cortex – This is the ventral segment of the frontal lobe which is involved in the cognitive process of decision-making. It is connected to the sensory and limbic system which mediate emotion and memory. In recent years, reports of pedophilic behavior resulting from damage or compression of this part of the frontal lobe by brain tumors, have been published in the medical literature.

Where Is Heaven And Hell?

Eternal Damnation

Soul And Biologic Body

"I have never seen the slightest scientific proof of the religious theories of heaven and hell, of future life for individuals, or of personal God." – **Thomas Edison (1847-1931), American inventor**

"Finding that no religion is based on facts and cannot be true, I began to reflect what must be the condition of mankind trained from infancy to believe in error." – **Robert Owen (1771-1858), a Welsh textile manufacturer, philanthropist, and social reformer**

"I don't want to believe. I want to know." – **Carl Sagan (1934-1996) – astronomer, astrophysicist, astrobiologist, cosmologist, and planetary scientist**

"Play hard, work hard, love hard…The bottom line for me is to live life to the fullest in the here-and-now instead of hope-for hereafter, and make every day count in some meaningful way and do something—no matter how small it is—to make the world a better place." – **Michael Shermer, founder and publisher, *Skeptic Magazine***

"I cannot believe in a God who wants to be praised all the time." – **Friedrich Nietzsche (1844-1900), German philosopher, post and cultural critic**

Religious parents teach their children that heaven is where good people go after death and they live a wonderful life forever and ever—and hell is where bad people go after death and they suffer extreme heat, endlessly. Simplistically, heaven is located above in the sky, while hell is located below the surface of the earth. Science tells us that above the earth and beyond are trillions of stars and various celestial objects, and below the earth's surface are decaying organic materials, tectonic plates, and a molten core of magnetic iron and various metals and minerals. Children are urged to pray and avoid committing sins to guarantee a place in heaven; otherwise, they go to hell—despite absence of physical evidence for the existence of either. These teachings, particularly the strong fear of going to hell, are quite powerful and compelling. When inculcated into the minds of innocent children, they become permanently retained within the limbic formation, particularly in the amygdala (along with its projections to the prefrontal cortex and hippocampus), where the instinct and emotion of fear are stored.

The ramifications of certain actions considered sinful, according to the Ten Commandments, can generate various psychiatric symptoms, ranging from anxiety, fear, and guilt to obsessive-compulsive behavior, and depression. Perhaps whoever devised this set of rules—God, gods, advanced ancient civilizations, or gods from outer space—were aware that the brain, just like any other organ, can be afflicted with various structural aberrations that can lead to the development of various personality and behavioral disorders. Therefore, whoever was involved in what appears to have been an intelligent intervention to create humans knew full well that these variations in personalities could lead to antagonism, hostilities, envy, and greed among humans, Hence, there was a need to temper the natural violent behavior of humans by formulating the mind-controlling Ten Commandments. Of course, for those with strong faith, this set of rules was all about Moses and his god, and no other.

Neurologically, it is difficult to understand how a certain human will go to hell or heaven for certain actions, knowing full well that behavior is mediated by several pools of neurons in their limbic system. Self-preservation, selfishness, lying, materialism, blaming others, jealousy, envy, resentment, abdication of self-responsibility, seeking the pain of others as a form of revenge, and sexual misconduct—all exist to varying degrees in all humans—and all are considered sinful acts and are therefore punishable by possible eternal damnation. Persons who are purely altruistic and truly kindhearted are theoretically bound to go to heaven. Realistically, however, all things considered, determining who will really go to heaven or to hell is difficult. Will confession and prayers lead to salvation? If the sinner goes to hell, why would God punish the object of His creation? Quite ironic, isn't it? An analogy can be made with the destruction of a computer and electronic gadgets if they fail to do what the owner wanted them to do after programming them.

According to the belief system of devout religious people, the soul is composed of the mind, will, and emotion and separates from the biologic body upon death of an individual. This soul, when it separates from the body of a good person, will go to heaven; otherwise, it will go to hell or somewhere in between. This is a simplistic belief among Christians, despite the absence of scientific evidence. The existence of the soul, at times used interchangeably with the spirit, is often dramatized and sensationalized in Hollywood movies, often reinforcing the belief that such a thing exists. Strangely, it is portrayed as a human-shaped transparent object, with a head and extremities, that can penetrate or pass through solid walls. Some cable television channels will even show programs that "prove" the soul can communicate with living relatives and friends. From the scientific standpoint, this is a gross display of disinformation or fake documentation of something without scientific basis, which misleads the gullible minds of the young and innocent and further cements their knowledge acquired through the process of indoctrination.

If a soul goes to hell, how is it possible to suffer in the eternal flame of hell when in fact the soul has no organic or inorganic constituents. Even if these constituents were present, they would eventually turn to ashes in a few minutes and no longer burn. Believers claim that the soul is composed of mind, will, and emotion, but those functions are mediated by the biological brain, specifically in the limbic system. How can these mental functions remain active when the brain dies? How can a soul carry out those mental functions? For those devout believers, nothing will ever change. Heaven and hell will forever exist—plain and simple—so believe what you were told by the ecclesiastical authorities, and stop asking any more questions. Period!!

The soul is believed to be created by God at the moment of conception or at a later date (this is, of course, conjectural). In most religions, the soul is the essence of a human being. The term soul was derived from Old English "sawol," meaning an immortal principle in man. The Christian concepts of body–soul originated with the ancient Greeks and were later acquired by the Christians. Aristotle described it as "the actuality of a body that has life." According to Plato, the soul is an independent entity, and it exists prior to its incorporation into the organic body. The real issue, however, is how the concept originated and what led the ancients to formulate the existence of something without demonstrable chemical constituents or something that could be perceived by special senses.

Are humans the only beings with souls? What about other living beings, such as lower forms of mammals and animals, parasites, bacteria, fungi, viruses, prions, and other microorganisms? If pathogenic microorganisms have souls, where will they go after being annihilated by antibiotics and after killing the animal or human host? What about animal predators, like lions, tigers, leopards, cheetahs, and hyenas, that hunt and kill weaker animals? If humans are the only beings with souls in the animal kingdom, was it unfair for God to single out humans alone to provide them with souls? How is it possible for the soul to control and regulate the 100 billion neurons, along with 10-fold more glial cells in the brain, not to mention the several million neurons in the spinal cord? What about the trillions and trillions of cells in the internal organs outside the central and peripheral nervous system? Thomas Edison (in *Do We Live Again?*) remarked, "My mind is incapable of conceiving such a thing as a soul. I may be in error, and man may have a soul, but I simply do not believe it."

> *"There is a good possibility, in fact, that the soul is a deeply rooted concept rather than reality—militant atheists would go even further and describe the soul as pure superstition."* – **Deepak Chopra, M.D., F.A.C.P. – world-renowned pioneer in integrative medicine and personal transformation**

Catholics are, in general, superstitious. The strong belief in the existence of the soul has led them to think that it sometimes comes back and shows itself to the relatives or friends it left behind. At times, the soul can appear in the form of a butterfly or any other animal, a sudden gust of wind, or the smell of a burning candle.

The frequency may vary from once a month to once a year or more frequently if the dead person had left behind an "unfinished project or unfulfilled promises." Posting blessed religious portraits, usually pictures of Jesus Christ and Virgin Mary, on the walls of houses or buildings for "protection" against evil is a common practice among Catholics. Exorcism was a centuries-old practice in Catholic religion during the Dark Ages. Inspired by a movie titled "The Exorcist " in 1973, it is still being practiced in some Catholic countries, particularly Brazil and Latin American countries. The legitimacy of the practice has been acknowledged by Pope Francis. It has been the stuff of fiction and horror movies. It is a religious or spiritual practice of "expelling" the devil or other spiritual entities from a person believed to be possessed. The purpose of the devil is to conquer the souls of humans. The practice of exorcism is endorsed and practiced by the Vatican, where several thousand cases have been "treated" by exorcism in the past several years.

To date, no studies have investigated the personality profiles of people "possessed' by the devil. How many had mental illnesses, like psychosis, personality disorder, and obsessive-compulsive disorder? How many had degenerative neurological diseases or neoplasms in the brain? How many had been evaluated by psychiatrists and/or neurologists, and underwent diagnostic procedures such as electroencephalograms, computerized and positron-emission tomography, and functional magnetic resonance imaging of the brain? As a freethinker and truth seeker, I find these to be important questions that cannot be ignored. In this world we live in, misinformation and disinformation have abounded since time immemorial, and the world has been this way to fit the ideological narrative of some powerful organized religious and political groups. It is unimaginable to think that endless fake information has been propagated to the lay public for thousands of years and was eventually and unfortunately incorporated into the neural fabric of innocent and scientifically unsophisticated people. Sad, but true.

Some claim that God—who is all-knowing, all-powerful, loving, and just—created everything, including trillions of stars billions of light years away from each other in the universe. Do other star systems have a history of Jesus Christ, Moses, God of the Old and New Testaments, Mary, Joseph, and the apostles? Will their creations include evil? Does evil exist in other star systems? If Satan is the symbol of evil, does that mean that Satan was created by God? Has anyone seen Satan? What nonbelievers find difficult to understand is why God would allow evil, which he created, to intimidate and defeat the good and the innocent. Glory to God in the highest.

CHAPTER 6

The Out-Of-Body Experience And Near-Death Experience

Myths And Facts

"Out-of-body flight 'really happens,' then—it is a real physical event, but only in the patient's brain and, as a result, in his subjective experience. The out-of-body state is, by and large, an exacerbated form of the dizziness that we all experience when our vision disagrees with our vestibular system, as on a rocking boat." **– Stanislas Dehaene, in "Consciousness and the Brain: Deciphering How the Brain Codes Our Thoughts"**

"Sometimes people don't want to hear the truth because they don't want their illusions destroyed." **– Friedrich Nietzsche**

Out-of-body experience (OBE) literally means seeing oneself from a distance outside the physical body. It has occurred in some people during cardiac arrest, near-drowning, electrolyte imbalance (as in dehydration), traumatic head injuries, epilepsy, migraine, vestibular disorders, and while under the influence of psychedelic drugs. Near-death experience (NDE), a form of OBE, has been reported by some people who were supposedly on the verge of "dying." While in this state, they have observed bright lights and strange figures and interpreted this as being in a strange place that seems to resemble "heaven". Thus, the concept of soul was born following reports of OBE and NDE by people who experienced this phenomenon. For the believers—professionals and nonprofessionals alike—it is living proof that God, soul, and heaven exist; however, to the skeptics and truthseekers, this phenomenon is simply a manifestation of a brain that is being irritated and stimulated due to a lack of blood supply and oxygen. In this situation, in a person who is deeply religious and has "implanted" the images of Jesus Christ and heaven in his or her parietal, temporal, and occipital lobes, these images can "reappear" during the state of OBE or NDE.

NDE, in my opinion, is a misnomer. Death is either sudden, as in people who die in an airplane crash, or slow, as in people dying from cancer, severe drug overdose, chronic obstructive pulmonary disease, severe congestive heart failure, or terminal liver or kidney disease, or those who sustain brain anoxia and become brain dead following a massive heart attack. A person who is terminally as a result of the above conditions passes through a stage of lethargy and obtundation, followed by coma and death. That person will not survive to tell their story. Realistically, there is no in-between. The word "death" in NDE is inappropriate, because the person in that situation is not dying per se; rather, the brain is "struggling" to acquire a blood supply and oxygen. In this situation, areas in the brain (i.e., the angular and supramarginal gyri and vestibulo-auditory centers—Figure 3), when subjected to metabolic or hypoxemic changes due to lack of nutrients or oxygen, will generate impulses that will result in the production of abnormal visuospatial images, including OBE. If the same person fails to be revived by cardiopulmonary resuscitation, he will then become either brain dead or totally dead—and there is no way that person will live to tell his NDE or OBE. Moreover, OBE has been reported in conditions that are not associated with dying, such as vestibular disorders, migraine, epilepsy, and effect of psychedelic drugs. In these situations, NDE is obviously not applicable and not appropriate.

The parietal lobe and its components are fascinating parts of the cerebral hemisphere. Together with the angular and supramarginal gyri, it controls visual and spatial awareness. The somesthetic component receives sensory projections from the thalamus and contralateral side of the body. A lesion in the parietal lobe will result in loss of position and passive movement; inability to localize touch, temperature, and pain stimuli applied to body surface; inability to distinguish the size, shape, and texture of objects; inability to recognize figures or numbers drawn on the skin; inability to draw geometric figures; defective two-point discrimination; and extinction of one side of the body during double simultaneous stimulation. At times, following a stroke, patients may become unaware of the paralyzed side of the body or even deny that it belongs to them. If asked to raise the paralyzed side, they will move their good arm. Blunted emotion is common. The patients may experience indifference to failure and may develop hallucinations of movements, along with illusions of visual and tactile stimuli. As discussed in this chapter, stimulation of the right, parietal, and temporal lobe junctions, where the angular, supramarginal, and vestibular-auditory gyri are located, has been reported to induce OBE.

Sleep is another physiologic process that can generate OBE. It has four to five stages. Stage 1 is the lightest stage of sleep and is associated with minimal slowing of brain wave activity. Muscle tone is retained during this stage. Soon, Stage 2 follows and is characterized by deeper sleep associated with the appearance of sleep spindles in electroencephalography (EEG). The deepest sleep occurs in Stages 3 and 4, during which time the EEG frequency becomes slow, and waking the individual can be very difficult. Stage 5 is usually called rapid eye movement sleep (also called paradoxical sleep). This is a unique stage of sleep in mammals and is characterized by rapid random eye movements, irregular breathing, and increased cardiac rate and blood pressure. The skeletal muscles become hypotonic or atonic. EEG traces may show lower voltage and mixed frequency patterns resembling wakefulness. This stage is most associated with vivid dreams, sexual arousal in both genders, facial twitchings, and vocal sounds and violent arm or leg movements at times. A total of 4–5 cycles of REM sleep may occur in a typical night. Stages 1–3 comprise 75–80% of total sleep. These stages are also called the non-REM sleep pattern.

The loss of muscle tone during REM sleep involves muscles from head to toes; in essence, the body is totally paralyzed. One animal study demonstrated that sleep paralysis is mediated by two neurotransmitters, gamma-aminobutyric acid and glycine, acting on the motor neurons in the spinal cord and brainstem (the pons and medulla). The paralysis is nature's way of protecting the body from injury when the individual experiences wild dreams and violent movements during the REM sleep stage.

Sleep paralysis may occur rarely while falling asleep but most commonly when emerging from or during the deep stage of REM sleep. It can be frightening, but it resolves immediately or spontaneously upon awakening. In some situations, REM sleep may occur in association with hypnagogic hallucinations, a condition that goes along with lucid dreams. Hallucinations may consist of a sensation of impending doom, fear, threat, a feeling of suffocation, and a sensation of spinning and floating, including OBE. They occur frequently in people with narcolepsy-cataplexy syndrome. One study (published in Neurology, 2006;66:1003-1009) performed by Dr. Kevin Nelson of the University of Kentucky in Lexington, reported that people with OBE are more prone to experience sleep paralysis. Dr. Nelson indicated that people who reported NDE may have an arousal system that allows REM sleep to "intrude" on wakefulness in times of distress. In a subsequent study, he and his colleagues interviewed 55 people who experienced "near-death" related to near drowning, heart attack, stroke, and vehicular accidents. Sixty percent had at least one episode of REM intrusion into their wakefulness. The hallucinations were visual and auditory and occurred while falling asleep, waking up from sleep, or during sleep paralysis. He added that the lights seen by people who reported OBE can be explained by retinal ischemia, similar to the visual symptoms that occur in retinal detachment and retinal migraine. Visual hallucinations have been reported in 60 percent of participants who experienced episodes of fainting. These phenomena can be attributed to a lack of blood flow to the brain and retina (Ann Neurol. 1994.36:233-237).

Investigators who conducted an earlier study of several hundred subjects with out-of-body experiences performed by a group of investigators from the University of California, Stanford University, and Wayne State University found a close association between OBE reporting and lucid dreams. They argued that all states of consciousness (sleeping or waking) are derived from the same basic brain functions that act to model the world based on perceptual maps in the somatosensory center of the brain (Levitan, L, LaBerge, S, DeGracia, DJ, et al. (1999). "Out-of-body experiences," dreams, and REM sleep. Sleep and Hypnosis. 1(3):186-196).

In recent years, OBE has been reported by patients undergoing neurosurgical procedures. An article published in New England Journal of Medicine, 2007;357:1829-1833, by the Department of Neurosurgery and Ear, Nose, and Throat, University Hospital Antwerp , Antwerp, Belgium, described a 63-year-old man who reported OBE while implanted electrodes at the temporoparietal junction were stimulated during the process of suppressing intractable tinnitus. To confirm this event, the patient underwent positron emission tomography, which demonstrated an activated area in the junction of the angular-supramarginal gyrus, an area that mediates multisensory integration combined with activation of a second area in the posterior part of the superior temporal cortex, a region associated with self-perception.

An interesting study conducted by A.M. Smith and C. Messier at the University of Ottawa described a subject who reported being able to reproduce somatosensory sensations that she experienced as her body moving outside of her physical body. Using functional MR imaging, the investigators demonstrated activations in the parietotemporal region (supramarginal gyri), left supplementary cortex, and cerebellum (Voluntary Out-of-Body Experience: An fMRI study. Published on line 2014 Feb 10.Doi:10.3389/fnhum.2014.00070). These results suggest that the extracorporeal experience reported by this subject represents an unusual type of kinesthetic imagery.

A few years later, OBE was reported in a patient undergoing an awake craniotomy for resection of low-grade glioma. The case was reported by the Department of Neurosurgery and Radiology, Erasmus Medical Center, Rotterdam, the Netherlands, in an article published in World Surgery, 92;586/e9-586.e13. Subsequent stimulation of the left temporoparietal junction induced OBE. Similarly, a patient who underwent awake craniotomy for epilepsy, performed by Wilder Penfield in 1941, reported OBE when the right superior temporal gyrus was stimulated. The patient did not have a history of OBE prior to surgery.

A prospective, observational study of 210 patients with dizziness reported a higher occurrence of OBE in 14% of patients when compared to age- and gender-matched controls without a history of dizziness (Lopez, C, Elziere, M., 2018. Out-of-body experience in vestibular disorders—A prospective study of 210 patients with dizziness. Cortex. 104:193-206). This is not surprising because of the proximity of the supramarginal and angular gyri to the auditory–vestibular center in the brain.

The brain is a truly fascinating organ in the human body. Unlike the stereotyped manifestations that occur when an extracranial organ is afflicted by a certain disease process, the brain may manifest myriad symptoms that usually mystify those who are not familiar with the science of neurology. Visual and auditory symptoms occur in a number of conditions, such as various hallucinations related to schizophrenia and psychedelic drugs, hypnagogic hallucinations related to REM sleep and narcolepsy syndrome, hallucinations and delirium in metabolic encephalopathy, and visual symptoms related to retinal disease and migraine, but other forms of cerebral phenomena also resemble hallucinations. These hallucinatory-like symptoms include palinopsia and palinacousis, both of which can be induced by neoplasm, stroke, vascular lesions, abscess, seizures, and medications (Palinopsia: Rare but ominous symptom of cerebral dysfunction, Neurosurgery. 1983;13:310-313). The word palinopsia is derived from the (Greek word "palin," which means "again" and "opsis," which means seeing. It is the perseveration or persistence of an image or seeing an image after the initial stimulus is removed. It is different from the physiological afterimage that occurs transiently after staring at a bright object. Palinacousis (acousis means hearing) has the same mechanism

(HandB Clin Neurol, 2015;129:457-467). One can only wonder how these visual and auditory phenomena were interpreted by the ancients. In all likelihood, they were probably considered works of the devil, divine events, or magical powers.

What are the implications of these visual and auditory phenomena, and how are they related to apparitions, miracles, OBE, NDE, and sinful acts? Quite likely, all these cerebral phenomena have occurred numerous times in the distant past, but obviously nobody knew their meaning or nature. However, based on the interpretations of these phenomena made by the ancients, they were considered supernatural, divine, works of evil, and devilish possession. Some people who reported these phenomena might have correlated them with or blamed them on sinful acts they had committed in the recent past. The ramifications of misinterpreting them as something divine or evil are obvious and will only reinforce the belief systems, such as the Christian religion, which has a basic foundation in which superstitions and belief in the afterlife are part of the social fabric.

Angular gyrus

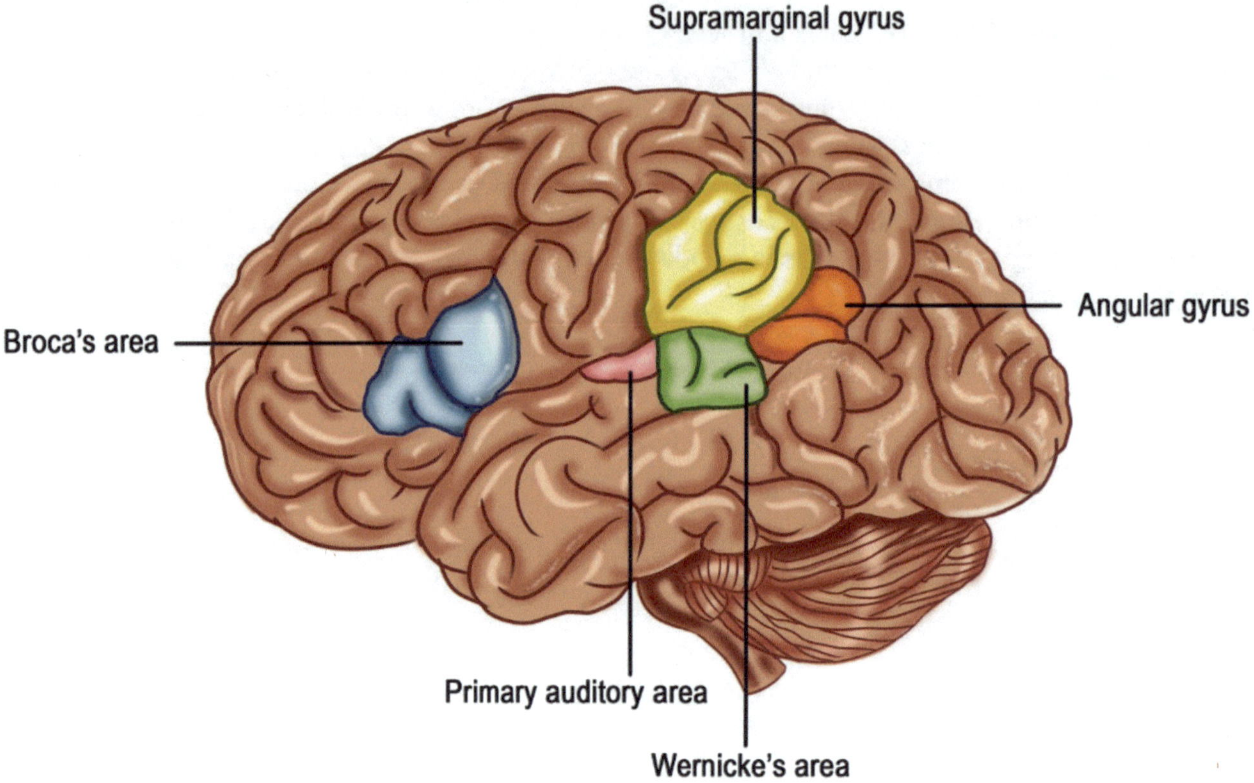

Angular and supramarginal gyri - These gyri are the lower segments of the parietal lobe. They have been implicated in the phenomenon of "out-of-body" including "near-death" experiences. They are essential for visuospatial awareness, and are involved in hallucinatory and illusory experiences.

CHAPTER 7

Confession, Sin And Repeat Offenders

Personality Characteristics Of Very Religious People

"It could be ventured to understand obsessive compulsive neurosis as the pathologic counterpart of religious development, to define neurosis as an individual religiosity; to define religion as a universal obsessive compulsive neurosis." – **Sigmund Freud (1856–1939), Austrian neurologist and founder of psychoanalysis**

"Cults recruit people by offering a counterfeit form of acceptance and purpose, which is also how religion operates. Like a cult, religion discourages questions and marginalizes those who fail to toe the line." – **Carl Jung (1878–1961), Swiss psychiatrist and psychotherapist**

"Science has eradicated small pox, can immunize against most previously deadly viruses, can kill most previously deadly bacteria. Theology has done nothing but talk of pestilence as the wages of sin." – **Richard Dawkins, author of *God Delusion***

"When they asked me what my religion was, I said I was Non-Delusional." – **atheist saying (www.geckoandfly.com)**

"For every player who credits God for the win, a player from the opposing team can logically blame God for the loss." – **Neil deGrasse Tyson, American astrophysicist and science communicator**

Growing up in the Philippines—a predominantly Catholic nation with a population of at least 70,000,000 million people when I left the country in 1971 (and now at least 100,000,000) whose citizens look up the sky and pray every day—was a riveting, anxiety-creating, guilt-producing, and confusing experience. People there attend church, join religious processions, and observe religious holidays. Bloodcurdling and gruesome religious festivals take place on Good Friday, where dozens of compunctious devotees re-enact Christ's sufferings by having their palms and feet nailed onto crosses by participants dressed as Roman centurions, after carrying the cross under the heat of the sun for a long distance or after self-flagellation using wooden whips. These practices are not endorsed by the Catholic Church, and obviously not advised by the medical profession. The belief in Jesus Christ is so strong among Christians and Catholics that they have developed animosity and hostility toward religious groups, particularly those of the Jewish faith, that deny the claim that he is the Messiah and the savior.

Despite the atrocities and abuses committed by the Spaniards and their clergy against the Filipinos from the time Ferdinand Magellan set foot on Philippine soil 500 years ago, the Philippines became the only Catholic nation in Asia. Its people are very religious—young and old, and rich and poor alike. Unfortunately, their religiosity is not rewarded by prosperity and good health. The gap between affluence and poverty continues to widen. Slums and squatter areas are commonplace, while the rich live in luxurious houses surrounded by concrete walls. The country remains economically behind other non-Catholic Asian nations. People go to confession and receive communion regularly, and yet crimes, graft, and corruption in the government are rampant. Poverty and death from natural disasters (typhoons, floods, earthquakes, and volcanic eruptions) have not been prevented by prayers. Children are often born out of wedlock. My father and his brothers, who memorized and could recite several passages in the Bible and went to confession and received communion several times a year, were philanderers and involved in many graft and corruption practices while working for the local government. One of my sisters, together with her children, made unfair and clandestine sales of our family inheritance properties in the Philippines to enrich themselves without my prior knowledge and consent. They entered the United States through sneaky legal maneuvering. Her husband was able to obtain disability benefits shortly after their arrival in the Golden State of California. They are the same people who go to church every Sunday, go to confession every year, receive communion every week, travel to several churches, and pray during the Lenten season. In essence, they are committing the sin of hypocrisy. They claim to believe in something, act in a different manner, and pretend to be what they are not.

Traditionally, Catholic authorities advise their members to go to confession once a year. At the conclusion of confession, the confessor is given penance by the priest. The penance consists of reciting the "Lord's Prayer," Hail Mary," and "Apostles' Creed," including praying the rosary, depending on the seriousness of the sins. Confession is followed by communion the following Sunday. After the rituals, the "sinners" feel refreshed and satisfied, and they are confident they will be rewarded a nice place in the afterlife. However, those who commit mortal sins are disqualified from receiving communion and are subject to eternal damnation, so to speak.

Unlike the Catholic religion, the Protestant denominations teach their followers to confess directly to God. Judaism advises its members to include their confession in the prayers they recite three times a day. Islam does not think man was born a sinner. Satan is considered the sinner because he urged Adam and Eve to eat the apple from the tree. According to Islamic teachings, there is no middleman or any intermediary person is needed to communicate with God. It makes sense, realistically speaking, because if God is omnipresent—any person can pray anywhere regardless of location or day of the week. However, if the followers do not congregate and pray during the holidays of obligation or during weekends, places of worship will lose financial support and become bankrupt, since money donations are collected during those days.

Many years ago, a dramatic and spectacular confession was shown on television. A televangelist who had committed adultery made a confession in front of several thousand congregants and television viewers. He was sobbing and crying loudly while asking God for forgiveness. His confession was followed by thunderous ovation and cheers from the faithful congregants, apparently signifying forgiveness. However, whether he was really forgiven by God is another matter.

The neuroscientific aspect of sin is practically unknown to a great majority of devout followers, including some professionals. When a person suffers from cancer or from an acute or chronic illness affecting the liver, heart, intestines, or other organs, the usual reaction by others is sympathy, sorrow, and compassion toward the affected individual. Similar reactions generally occur for persons suffering from stroke, malignant tumor, or degenerative disorders of the brain. However, a person suffering from psychosis and various personality disorders who commits a sinful act is treated differently. Part of the reason is a lack of knowledge about the neuroscientific aspects of human behavior and emotion, which are regulated and controlled by various interconnecting neural networks in the limbic system.

The neural networks, along with various neurotransmitters, have a great degree of variability, which can explain why some people have different personality traits and intelligence. Some people react to stress in a different fashion. Some can take jokes and some cannot. Some have better memory and intellect. Some are optimistic, and some are pessimistic and cynical. Some are extroverted, and some are introverted. Some are temperamental and impulsive, and some are restrained. Some are gullible, and some tend to be skeptical or resistant to indoctrination. Radiologically, some may show differences in the gray and white matter volume, resulting in changes in sexual orientation. Some may show findings in the orbitofrontal cortex of the cerebrum and develop a perverted sexual preference or attraction, and some may become overly sexually aggressive. Be that as it may, any person who harbors certain aberrant neural connections in the brain is treated with disdain and indifference, not with sympathy and understanding. People who go to confession can regularly commit the same transgression and ask for forgiveness again and again. They feel refreshed and elated each time after "serving time" for the penance they received from a priest—who, incidentally, maybe a sinner himself or possibly a pedophile. This is one of the ironies and hypocrisies of religion.

> *"The inhabitants of the earth are of two sorts: those with intelligence but no religion, and those with religion but no intelligence"* – **Abu al-'ala al-Ma'arri (973-1057), Arab philosopher, poet, and writer**

Is there a distinct personality that characterizes religious people? Are religious people generally less intelligent? Are intelligent people more inquisitive and analytical? Is intelligence relative? According to the Oxford Dictionary, "intelligence is having the ability to understand or identify unfamiliar or difficult circumstances, respond to them and deduce solutions." It involves the ability to effectively communicate verbally and nonverbally, the ability to discern the differences in emotion and moods, and the ability to offer new ideas and entertain multiple perspectives. Intelligent people have a higher degree of openness and are more percipient. They are more likely to keep going, acquire new knowledge, and challenge mainstream social practices. Notably, some professionals, such as physicians, remain adherent to their beliefs and faith, despite their knowledge of biological sciences. This is an amazing testament to the power of the religious indoctrination process initiated during childhood. These are the same people who are proficient in several science subjects but, at the same time, instinctively accept an institution based on a belief system that was acquired from ancient people, people with no concept of science. Ironic, isn't it?

One big difference separates those (professionals and some laypersons) with intelligence and religion, and those with intelligence (some neuroscientists, astronomers, and astrophysicists) but without religion. The difference lies in the presence or absence of obsessive-compulsive behavior (OCB), a condition that denotes a compulsion to perform certain stereotyped actions repetitively to alleviate persistent fears or unpleasant and unwelcome thoughts. Some people may spend minutes or hours—or they may consume the whole day—performing acts that alleviate those intrusive thoughts. Religious OCB is seen in many cultures. A person with religious OCB has an overwhelming urge to pray and ask for forgiveness to "wash" their soul and guarantee a place in heaven. A particular pathologic guilt about moral or religious issues is called scrupulosity, or sometimes "religious obsessive-compulsive disorder," a condition I have personally observed among many downtrodden Filipinos. This phenomenon has its roots in years of oppression and subjugation of traits suffered under Spanish rule. It is a pathologic preoccupation with sin and the fear and guilt associated with it. It is a debilitating concern about morality—a product of rigorous religious indoctrination during childhood. Whether OCB is due to innate abnormal neural networks in the limbic system or something acquired and nurtured through repetitive religious teachings and epigenetic mechanisms remains an open issue. The neuroanatomical and neurochemical aspects of OCB are detailed in Chapter 2.

I am not doubting the intellectual capacity of my classmates, but their strong and eerily tenacious religious convictions are quite remarkable. Most of them spent at least thirteen years obtaining a premedical and medical education, including postgraduate training in this multi-cultural and multi-faith society known as the United States of America, to master the science of medicine. Am I saying that my classmates have religious OCB? Based on my association with them during our years in medical school, including analysis of e-mail exchanges in the past ten years, I must say, unmistakably and empathetically, that they are indeed religiously indoctrinated and suffering from varying degrees of religious OCB—and they are not even aware of it or simply deny it. A great majority of them are retired, and understandably may have lost some of their medical skills, but not their religious beliefs and knowledge of the Bible that they acquired during their childhood. This is not surprising when one applies the law that was hypothesized by Theodule Ribot (1839-1916), a French psychologist, who stated that "there is a time gradient in retrograde amnesia, so that recent memories are more likely to be lost than the more remote memories" – en .wikipedia.org/wiki/Ribot's _law

Besides religious OCB, certain other traits distinguish religious people. Some of them believe that being methodical, highly self-disciplined, high-achieving, cautious, trustworthy, compassionate, honest, forgiving, and compliant is closely associated with religiosity. Possession of these traits is perhaps driven by the reward of eternal life. Anecdotally, however, I have met and have been associated with compatriots, medical colleagues, and patients who possess the above traits but are not religious, and consider themselves agnostics or atheists. Conversely, there are some religious people who are not generous, cheat on their taxes, and make obscene profits from their business firms—the same people who go to confession regularly, year after year, and feel good after serving their penance. Some politicians who claim they are not supposed to hate anybody because they are Catholics are the same people who go after their political rivals and harass them relentlessly so they can stay in power, the power they use to influence big business companies. Many are suspected of having insider trading knowledge in the stock market and to have enriched themselves quite remarkably. Will these politicians be rewarded with a cozy place in the afterlife?

> *"Faith: not wanting to know what is true."* – **Friedrich Nietzsche**
>
> *"Faith can be very dangerous and deliberately to implant it into the vulnerable mind of an innocent child is a grievous wrong."* – **Richard Dawkins, author of "God Delusion"**

Thou Shalt Not Kill And Instinct To Survive: Animals Killing Their Prey, Microbials Killing Their Animal Hosts, Scientists Sacrificing Animals In Laboratory Experimentations, Soldiers Killing Enemy Soldiers, And Explorers Who Killed Native Inhabitants While Spreading Christianity

Capital Punishment

Women's Rights And Termination Of Pregnancy

"God said, 'Thou shalt not kill'—does the theft of a little money make it quite all right for us to do so? If it's said that this commandment applies only to illegal killing, what's to prevent human beings from similarly agreeing among themselves to legalize certain types of rape, adultery, or perjury? Considering that God has forbidden us even to kill ourselves, can we really believe that purely human arrangements for the regulation of mutual slaughter are enough, without any divine authority, to exempt executioners from the sixth commandment? Isn't that like saying that this particular commandment has no more validity than what human laws allow it?—in which case the principle can be extended indefinitely, until in all spheres of life human beings decide just how far God's commandments may conveniently be observed." **– Thomas Moore (1779-1852), Irish writer, poet, and lyricist**

"The very emphasis of the commandment: 'Thou shalt not kill,' makes it certain that we are descended from an endlessly long chain of generation of murderers, whose love of murder was in their blood as it is perhaps in ours." **– Sigmund Freud (1856-1939), Austrian neurologist and founder of psychoanalysis**

"'Thou shalt not kill' does not apply to murder of one's own kind only, but to all living beings and this commandment was inscribed in the human breast long before it was proclaimed from Sinai." **– Leo Tolstoy (1828), Russian author, "On Life and Essays on Religion"**

"Thou shalt not kill." This sixth commandment is brief and to the point, but unfortunately vague and unclear. It was given to Moses by God on Mount Sinai, along with the other nine. Unfortunately, no witnesses were present to describe what Moses actually saw or heard. When God arrived, Mount Sinai was reportedly covered with smoke. The whole mountain and the ground below were shaking. There was a "trumpet" sound that blasted louder and louder. There was "thunder and flashes of lightning" as the "Lord" descended from the sky. God advised Moses to tell the people not to climb the mountain and that they must not look upon the "face" of the God. After 40 days, Moses descended from the mountain carrying the Ten Commandments. He looked older, his face and skin shone, and his hair was long and white. Some researchers have speculated that that Moses possibly had an encounter with extraterrestrial beings and might have been exposed to radiation emitted from their extraterrestrial space vehicle. At this time, believers cannot offer any explanations as to why the arrival of God was heralded by light, thunder, smoke, and shaking of the ground. This event took place at the time when human intelligence was far below today's intellectual level, not to mention the total lack of technology and science during that time. For some reason, the God that spoke to Moses on Mount Sinai has never been seen since, and certainly not by modern humans, to elaborate the commandments further.

The lack of clarity of the sixth commandment has generated numerous questions as to its exact meaning and its applicability in modern times. The commandment did not specify killing other living beings, such as insects, fish, various microorganisms, plants, and vegetation. In subsequent years, religious people tried to put a spin on how to elaborate the meaning of the commandment. Humans are allowed to kill animals for food, but murdering fellow humans is morally condemned and punishable by eternal damnation, and legally punishable through incarceration and/or capital punishment. Are humans allowed to kill lower forms of animals for recreation? If so, did God specify that in the commandment? Obviously, he did not. What about stronger animals killing their weaker prey for food? This is probably allowable for survival, but weaker animals have the right to live too. Morally, who is accountable for sacrificing animals for the sake of science, the ultimate aim of which, understandably, is to improve future healthcare? If God is fair, why would he allow this to happen to helpless defenseless animals like Sprague Dawley rats, guinea pigs, monkeys, cats, and dogs? In some towns in a very religious nation like the Philippines, domesticated dogs are killed and eaten. Roosters, armed with razor-sharp blades securely attached to their legs, fight to death in lucrative gambling sports in almost all towns and cities in that country. Where are the animal rights activists? Unfortunately, they are helpless and unable to act to save the roosters because of the notoriously corrupt political system in this fervent Catholic nation. Yes, that's correct—very religious and yet corrupt.

Killing of humans evolved from using stones and wood, followed by using sharp metals to express anger against fellow humans. Today, humans die from bullets, high-speed missiles, and devastating bombs when they kill each other for various reasons. The end of humanity may not be far off on the horizon if an all-out war erupts among powerful nations that have nuclear bombs, the bombs that killed thousands and thousands of Japanese citizens during World War II.

During times of war, young soldiers are sent to the front to fight and kill enemy soldiers. If a soldier killed hundreds of enemy soldiers (each one married and a father with several children), would he be allowed to confess and receive communion? Will he be allowed to enter the hypothetical heaven, or will he be sent down to hypothetical hell?

In Chapter 13 of *A Neurologist's Daring Escape from the Steel Cage of Religion: A Long and Arduous Personal Journey to Reality*, I discussed the reality that religion is an inherently violent institution. It is indeed ironic that millions were murdered, all in the name of religion, the religion that carries and spreads the sixth commandment, "thou shalt not kill." Explorers and missionaries forcibly introduced Christianity onto native inhabitants of the lands they supposedly discovered, but subsequently murdered any inhabitants who refused to accept their religion. It is worth repeating in this book that millions of Jews were killed by Adolph Hitler, a Catholic, during World War II and that millions of native inhabitants of the Americas were killed by Spanish explorers, including Christopher Columbus, as they spread their Christian religion. Were Hitler or these explorers and missionaries rewarded with a cozy place in heaven, or were their souls sent down to the eternal flame of hell? Mohandas Gandhi (1869-1948), in *The Degeneration of Belief,* remarked. "The most heinous and the cruelest crimes of which history has record have been committed under the cover of religion or equally noble motives." Other documented accounts of atrocities committed by Christians against other religious groups are listed in Chapter 9 of this book.

Whoever (God or advanced beings) gave Moses the Ten Commandments knew full well that humans, in general, are inherently aggressive and violent; hence, the mind-controlling nature of the commandments. Unfortunately, the rules were all simplistic and raised more questions than answers. If those commandments were handed to somebody similar to Moses during this modern age of scientifically and technologically savvy humans, that person would perhaps be bombarded with questions to clarify each commandment. For example, the sixth commandment is broad and subject to various interpretations, but it did not specifically mention termination of pregnancy, also known as abortion, at the time it was given to Moses. Perhaps it is possible that details about this commandment were lost in history and nowhere to be retrieved. Subsequently, however, modern religious humans tried to make further clarifications and re-structuring of the commandments, which then led to all actions ending a human life being included on death row, including ending the lives of the unborn.

When does a fetus become human? According to Christian teaching, the moment the male cell unites with female cell, a human life is born—and terminating it is a mortal sin. Through the use of ultrasound, waves of the fetal heartbeat can be detected as early as three weeks after fertilization, although the other organs have not fully developed. At some time during the 5th–6th weeks of pregnancy, the sonogram can get demonstrate the heartbeat. "Quickening," the term that indicates the first fetal movement, occurs during the 16th and 22nd week of pregnancy. It is an exciting time, especially for the mother-to-be, and is a sign of baby's health. However, the timing of the termination of a pregnancy is quite controversial. Some advocates of abortion maintain that pregnancy can be terminated before the fetus develops a heartbeat or before it develops a human form. With few exceptions, Christians oppose abortion at any stage of pregnancy.

When does a soul (if there is such a thing) begin to be incorporated into the biologic body? Does it happen when the spermatozoon enters the ovum? When the fetal heartbeat begins? When fetal movements occur? If a child is born without a brain (a condition termed "anencephaly"), does it have a soul? Without the brain, that child will never develop higher intellectual faculties. Will the soul of that child ever perceive anything neurologically after the death of the biological body? Realistically, an anencephalic child can only function at the level of the brainstem, meaning that the child cannot synthesize the degree and nature of the impulses at an intellectual level because of the absence of the cerebrum. All reactions are automatic (reflex reactions) and are not purposeful. Therefore, if the soul is located in the cerebrum and the limbic system, an anencephalic child should have no soul, and yet it can still move, albeit not purposefully. What will the soul of an aborted fetus look like during the first trimester or before it assumes a human form? If a soul was derived from a mentally retarded person, is that soul also retarded? What about the soul of a person who died of PD: will that soul also have a tremor? Is there a demented soul that separates from a person who dies of Alzheimer's disease or Lewy Body Dementia? Are the souls of Albert Einstein, Carl Sagan, and Stephen Hawking geniuses?

The issue of termination of pregnancy has been politicized by people from all walks of life, particularly by various members of the media outlets since its legalization in 1973, which was later overturned in a landmark decision by the Supreme Court in 2022 The intersection between women's rights and the sixth commandment has generated a severe divisive issue in U.S. politics, a hotly contested issue that exposed the contradictions and ironies in the practice of democracy and religion (particularly Catholic-based advocates) in this country—women's rights to control their bodies and religious rights to protect the lives of the innocent unborn. There appears to be a general unanimity in the decision-making process from both camps when the life of a pregnant mother is in danger or when the pregnancy is the result of incest or rape. Outside of these circumstances, things have become controversial and contentious. If the sixth commandment is to be followed, will the soul of women (including the soul of the health care providers that performed the abortion) who committed abortion for no other reasonable indications go to hell?

The instinct (or right) to survive began as soon as life appeared on the planet Earth 4.5 billion years ago (or a mere 6000 years, according to believers in the supernatural). This instinct is present in both animal and plant kingdoms. From single cells to multicellular organisms, the instinct to live and survive is part of life. Some microbes have to invade and disrupt the vital functions of their animal or human hosts to survive, but to the detriment of the latter's health and survival, unless antimicrobial medication is administered. The hierarchy of strength is well exhibited in Africa, where the strong predators stalk their weaker prey, kill, and eat them. Leaders of hostile and rogue countries continue to intimidate their weaker neighboring countries, and millions die in the ensuing wars, Many years ago, a religious classmate, a biblical expert, told me that all living beings in this world have a soul. One can only imagine, after the formation of the Earth 4.5 billion years ago (or 6000 years ago) and the billions of human beings that have been born and died on this planet, how overcrowded heaven and hell must be—full of "good and bad" souls, respectively—by now. On the other hand, hell will be empty if all sinners are forgiven. Conversely, heaven will be a boring place if all "bad" humans are sent down to hell.

Some people with major depressive disorder may lose the instinct to survive and commit suicide owing to impairments of the serotonin neurotransmitter system and abnormality in the neural circuitry in their hypothalamus, pituitary, and adrenal glands. Suicide, which is a form of killing, is considered a mortal sin. If those depressed people commit suicide due to neurochemical abnormality and/or paradoxical and unfortunate adverse side effects of anti-depressant medications, will their souls go to hell? Clearly, it is not fair to send the souls of mentally ill people to hell. Believers have no clear answers for this issue. What about suicide bombers who kill thousands of innocent lives in the name of religion? Will their souls be sent to heaven by their god to have sex with several virgins? Or to hell by the god of the dead people?

The term "capital punishment," also known as the death penalty, describes the killing of a person for serious crimes committed against another person, but it is a controversial issue in some countries and states. Serious crimes, called capital crimes or offenses, include murder and rape. They also include sexual abuse of minors, terrorism, aircraft hijacking, war crimes, genocide, treason, espionage, sedition, attempt to overthrow a government, aggravated robbery, kidnapping, drug trafficking, and drug possession. Execution of a person convicted of a capital crime is carried out by lethal injection, electrocution, gassing, or firing squad. In the past—and still in some countries—criminals were executed by hanging, stoning, shooting, burning at the stake, or boiling alive. Some people believe that capital punishment is cruel and inhumane, and they would prefer a life sentence with no chance of parole, along with restitution paid to the victim's relatives. Public perception, including the opinion of some authorities, is that the death penalty may not be very effective at deterring crime. Imposing a death penalty on a person wrongfully accused and convicted is an obvious and gross miscarriage of justice. Since recidivism is always a threat among violent criminals, either death or life in prison would lock criminals away from society.

Most nations have abolished capital punishment, but some countries retain the practice. These countries include China, India, some parts of the United States, Singapore, Indonesia, Pakistan, Bangladesh, Nigeria, Egypt, Saudi Arabia, Iran, Japan, and Taiwan. Capital punishment was legal in Vatican City between 1929 and 1969, but was reserved for attempted assassination of the Pope. However, executions were carried out elsewhere in the Papal States for a variety of offenses. The death penalty was supported by early Catholic theologians, such as St. Augustine and Thomas Aquinas, who argued that the punishment was supported by the scripture and was no way contrary to the sixth commandment. In 2018, Pope Francis declared that the death penalty was inadmissible because "it is an attack on the inviolability and dignity of the person." Some American conservatives are in favor of the death penalty and yet they are opposed to abortion. This is the opposite of what some American progressives stand for. This is clearly a conundrum in politics and religion in the multi-ethnic, multi-racial, and multi-faith country known as the United States of America. If killing is a sin, where will the souls of those who support the death penalty go?

Let us pray. God, please help the people on Earth clarify your sixth commandment, and please do not confuse the minds of the people you created. Amen.

Anachronism

Is A Perfect Society Possible And Viable?

Must Violence And Peace Exist Together To Maintain Checks And Balances?

Elimination Of Religious Indoctrination

"The ideal society can be described, quite simply, as that in which no man has the power of means to coerce others" – **Edward Abbey (1929-1989), American author and essayist**

"Religious dogma creates a perfect fertilizer for the weed of hypocrisy" – **Steve Maraboli, internet radio commentator, motivational speaker, and author of *Life, the Truth and Being Free***

"Is God willing to prevent evil, but not able? Then he is not omnipotent. Is he able, but not willing? Then he is malevolent. Is he both able, and willing? Then whence cometh evil? Is he neither able nor willing? Then why call him God?" – **Epicurus (34–270 BC), ancient Greek philosopher and sage**

"I am absolutely convinced that religion is the main source of hatred in this world" – **Christopher Hitchens (1949-2011), British-American orator and columnist, and author of *God is Not Great: How Religion Poisons Everything***

"On terms of history, Christianity is a relatively new religion. Just because it is popular today doesn't mean it will continue to have supporters and followers in the next thousand years. Atheism transcends religion, and at the end of the day, science is the only true that atheists believe in" – **Richard Dawkins, author of *God Delusion***

The Merriam-Webster dictionary defines anachronism as "something that is out of place in terms of time or chronology." The Free Dictionary defines it as "something out of its proper or chronological order, especially a person or practice that belongs to an earlier time." Christianity, which is just a little over 2000 years old, is an Abrahamic monotheistic religion derived from the life of Jesus Christ and his teachings, all recorded by hearsay without factual documentation. It is based on the Bible as sacred scripture, and professed by Eastern, Roman Catholic, and Protestant bodies. Others, however, have different opinions about the Bible. According to Bart D. Ehrman (March 25, 2011), "Many of the books of the New Testament were written by people who lied about their identity, claiming to be a famous apostle—Peter, Paul, or James. In modern parlance, that is a lie" (https://www.huffpost.com/entry/the-bible-telling-lies-to_b_840301). Here's an excerpt from the book titled *The Bible Fraud*, authored by Tony Bushby. "The Jewish records of the Rabbis are of extreme importance in determining Gospel origins and the value of the church presentation of the virgin birth story of Jesus Christ. A common appellation for Jesus in the Talmud was Yeshu'a ben Panthera, an allusion to the widespread Jewish belief during the earliest centuries of the Christian era that Jesus was the result of an illegitimate union between his mother and a Roman soldier named Tiberius Julius Abdes Panthera." Here's another excerpt from a book titled *The Christ Conspiracy: The Greatest Story Ever Sold*, authored by Acharya S. "There is basically no textual evidence of the existence of Jesus Christ other than forged biblical books and epistles." Despite the many questions brought up to authenticate the veracity of the gospel story and its main character, Jesus Christ, a religion was born out of the many controversies surrounding the true identity of the so-called son of God.

There are approximately 2.3 billion Christians in the world, making Christianity the largest religious institution in the world. The three largest Christian populations are found in the Americas and Europe. The third largest Catholic population in the world is found in the Philippines, the only Christian nation in Asia, with an estimated current population of at least 100,000,000. Protestant Christianity, introduced by the Americans in 1898 after the Spanish-American war, and Islam comprise the minority religions in that country.

Several years ago, when I revealed to my classmates during our e-mail exchanges that I was (and still am) nonreligious and a nonbeliever, I was instantaneously ostracized, vilified, and branded a sinner destined and guaranteed to go to hell. Some clandestinely urged others to cut off or ignore any form of communication with me. Most of my classmates are bible "experts," but they have remarkably meager knowledge of neurological sciences—a major issue that makes our thinking processes several light years apart. Even though I was born and raised in a very religious family and "educated" in religion in two parochial schools—and later became a neurologist—I was courageous enough (and fortunate) to acquire knowledge in investigative and alternative disciplines, such as archeoastronomy, atheism, and agnosticism, despite the threat of eternal damnation. Additional knowledge in medical genetics opened up a new perspective in my life and made me broadminded, farsighted, and a freethinker. The education and knowledge I acquired from these disciplines enabled me to escape from the powerful grip of religion.

The effects of religion on the human brain are astonishing. The power of indoctrination, especially when initiated during childhood, is bound to become permanently cemented into the neural fabric of the limbic system, and no amount of rehabilitation can reverse it. This is the reality that believers fail or refuse to recognize and accept. Even professionals, including physicians, can be hoodwinked, and their thinking process "frozen" in time. Christianity, strictly speaking, is anachronism derived from the ancient world 2000 years ago. It is a compilation of scripture written by superstitious, naïve, and gullible prehistoric people several thousand years ago before the advent of science. The teachings of religion are full of contradiction, hypocrisies, ironies, and paradoxes, but believers always find ways to twist and spin the issues to serve and defend their faith and belief system that were nurtured and cultivated by the powerful compulsive thought and threat of eternal damnation if they abandon the faith.

From the birth of Christianity 2000 years ago until the 14th century, everything about the religion was all about blind belief in authority. It is called faith—a refusal to know the truth and a compulsion to ignore science. Thousands and thousands of natives were murdered by explorers and missionaries because of their refusal to adopt the Christian religion or convert to Christianity. From the 14th century to the 17th century, the fervent period of European cultural, artistic, political, and economic advancements developed. This period is called the "Renaissance"—from Darkness (war, ignorance, famine, microbial pandemics) to Light (cultural, intellectual, and scientific advances). The renaissance started in Florence, Italy, when various writers, artists, and politicians decided to participate in an intellectual and artistic revolution. Pioneering and innovative Renaissance intellectuals during this period, to name a few, include the famous polymath Leonardo da Vinci (1452–1519), Rene Descartes (1596–1650), Galileo (1564–1642), Nicolaus Copernicus (1473–1543), Machiavelli (1469–1527), William Shakespeare (1564–1616), and Michelangelo (1475–1564).

Over the past three hundred years, the wave of civilization began to drift away from authoritarian (kings and emperors) and clergy rules toward democracy, secularism, and plurality. This shift was inspired by various intellectuals who began using reason and rationalization of religious events, particularly miracles and apparitions, that had been interpreted as divine and supernatural by the religiously indoctrinated. They began to question the validity of these events, including the existence of heaven and hell. Finally, in 18th century, an English-born American political activist, philosopher, and political theorist by the name of Thomas Paine (1737–1809) wrote a best-selling book titled *The Age of Reason*, published in three parts in 1794, 1795, and 1807. He argued for the philosophical position of deism that challenged institutionalized religion and the legitimacy of the Bible. He advocated reason in place of revelation, exposed corruption in the church, and advocated the rejection of miracles. He also considered the Bible an ordinary piece of literature, rather than a divinely inspired book. He also wrote two very influential pamphlets, *Common Sense* (1776) and *The American Crisis* (1776–1783), at the start of American revolution and helped inspire the patriots to declare independence from Great Britain in 1776.

Here are some of Paine's famous quotes about religion (excerpt from *A Neurologist's Daring Escape from the Steel Cage of Religion: A Long and Arduous Journey to Reality,* Lazaro, R., Peppertree Press, Chapter 8, 2022):

"To argue with a person who has renounced the use of reason is like administering medicine to the dead."

"My country is the world, and my religion is to do good."

"Of all tyrannies that affect mankind, tyranny in religion is the worst."

"The Bible is such a book of lies and contradictions; there is no knowing which part to believe or whether any."

"Belief in a cruel God makes a cruel man."

"It would be more consistent that we call the Bible the work of a demon than the word of God. It is a history of wickedness that has served to corrupt and brutalize mankind."

"Priests and conjurors are of the same trade."

"The Christian religion is a parody on the worship of the sun, in which they put a man called Christ in the place of the sun, and pay him the adoration originally paid to the sun."

"All the tales of miracles, with which the Old and New Testament are filled, are fit only for impostors."

"Each of those churches show certain books, which they call revelation, or the word of God. The Jews say their word of God was given by God to Moses face-to-face; the Christians say their word of God came by divine inspiration; and the Turks say that their word of God (the Koran) was brought by an angel from heaven. Each of those churches accuses the other of unbelief, and for my own part, I disbelieve them all."

The Age of Reason (or Enlightenment) has become the turning point and decisive moment in the history of mankind. It shone a bright light on the dark side of the believers' visual field, enabling them to develop new perspectives in science, morality, and politics, and to obtain maximum individual development. As a result, humans have come to realize that religions, particularly Christianity, are beset with contradictions and hypocrisies and are often the source of conflict. Sin, as defined by the Bible and Christian teachings, is influenced by self-preservation and ego and is corrupted by political affiliation and racial allegiance. The present society we now live in, where money controls everything, creates an environment that turns sinners who regularly go to confession into repeat offenders.

With continued advances in science, the landscape of religion in the US has changed quite remarkably in the past years. In telephone interviews conducted by the PEW Research Center in 2018 and 2019, 65% of American adults identified themselves as Christians, down by 12% over the previous 10 years. Protestants have experienced significant losses of congregation members. In this age of technology, the modern generation wants answers for everything, answers available at their fingertips and more likley their thumbs and smartphone now. They question the reliability and usefulness of prayers. Mass and sermons are boringly routine. Reports of priests, so-called men of God, charged with sexual molestation of children are quite disconcerting and ironic. Televangelists, committing fraud and adultery and pretending they can heal sick people, are disturbing and distressing. They close their eyes, pray, and beg for money. I must say, however, that there are some televangelists who are honest, honorable, trustworthy, and deserve to be called men of the God of their religions.

Even this long after Moses received the Ten Commandments in 1440 BC, humans all over the world continue to commit so-called sinful acts, which are either venial or mortal sins—and there are myriads of them. Actions, thoughts, and words considered selfish, harmful, shameful, and disruptive are equated with rejection of God. It is almost impossible for any human to be totally free of sin. It is clear that these commandments are all about mind control. The redundancy of the commandments is noteworthy. This was originally brought up by the late standup comedian, George Carlin (1937–2008), born and raised as a Catholic in New York City. According to Carlin, the commandments should be trimmed down to two as follows: "Thou shalt always be honest and faithful "and "Thou shalt try real hard not to kill anyone, unless of course, they pray to a different invisible man than the one you pray to."

It is quite appalling that, to this day, sinful acts are considered spiritual, and people totally ignore the neuroscientific aspects of human behavior. Simplistically, the believers assert that sin goes against God and his ways, but to the freethinkers and nonbelievers, the two words—sin and God—should not even exist. Broad estimates of those who do not believe in a supernatural deity range from 500 to 750 million people worldwide, the majority of whom reside in Asia and the Pacific, while the remainder reside in Europe, North America, Latin America, the Caribbean, sub-Saharan Africa, the Middle East, and North Africa. If not believing in God is considered a mortal sin, will these millions of people go to hell? What if these people did not kill anybody or commit suicide, were friendly, did not commit fraud, adultery, and perjury, and did not cheat on their taxes? Will their souls still go to hell? If they go to hell, why does God punish the objects of his own creation just because they did not believe in his existence?

Is a perfect society possible and viable? Depending on which side of the belief fence you are sitting on—creation, intelligent intervention by extraterrestrials, or fortuitous sequelae of the "Bing Bang"—humans never experience totally peaceful and pleasant events in their lifetime. Love and hate, peace and war, agreement and disagreement, friendship and hostility, and loyalty and treachery always occur and balance each other. It appears that a natural "ecology" exists in human behavior without which life can be either boring, tedious, and uninteresting or exciting, intriguing, and thought-provoking. In nature, humans and plants must coexist or the former will not survive without oxygen and the latter without carbon dioxide—and no life can exist on this planet without nitrogen, carbon, and hydrogen together with various minerals, metals, and trace elements. Advances in science, designed to maintain health and increase human longevity and to explore and explain the mysteries and the unknowns of the past and future, are counterbalanced by death due to wars, famine, and natural disasters and by faith-based religious education.

> *"Anyone who attempts to construe a personal view of God which conflicts with church dogma must be burned without pity."* – **Pope Innocent III, greatest single pre-Nazi mass murderer, 1209**

> *"It was even possible for the most venerated patriarchs of the church, like St. Augustine and St. Thomas Aquinas, to conclude that heretics should be tortured (Augustine) or killed (Aquinas)"* – **Sam Harris, neuroscientist, philosopher, and author of "The End of Faith" and "Free Will"**

> *"I don't ridicule religion, it ridicules itself"* – **Bill Maher, comedian and television host**

The Cambridge English Dictionary defines indoctrination as "the process of repeating an idea or belief to someone until they accept it without criticism or question." It is a process of inculcating a person or group of people to accept a set of beliefs, usually a partisan or sectarian principle, without question or reservation. Coercion and fear of going to hell, and an adage that says, "believe just in case but because there is nothing to lose but a lot to gain if God exists," are powerful messages, especially when delivered to children. Once this process is completed and successfully implanted into their limbic systems, the effect is either long-lasting or permanent. Recitation of "Lord's Prayer," "Hail Mary," and "Apostles' Creed," including praying the rosary after a confession, praying before dinner and before going to bed, and repeated sermons delivered by the priest on Sundays and religious holidays, are classic examples of indoctrination, aka brainwashing.

Is this world better without religion? Is there anything wrong with teaching children what is right and what is wrong, and what is legal and what is illegal, without amalgamating the teachings with a supernatural but invisible deity? If parents forcibly instill religious ideology into the brains of their children, should the children be made aware of the contradictions, hypocrisies, ironies, and paradoxes in religion to enable them to make their own decisions and choices? Unfortunately, the whole idea of indoctrination is to emphasize the positive and eliminate the negative. The process is easily accomplished in children, similar to the religious indoctrination of primitive and naïve societies of ancient civilizations who did not possess any knowledge of science and never had the opportunity to question the powerful religious authorities. Everything was all about mind control.

The atrocities and victims of the Christian faith are simply too numerous to discuss in detail. It is appalling that many devout believers are not aware of the way Christianity was spread and forcibly shoved down the throats of those people who refused to adopt the religion. Thousands of pagans, priests, and children were slain between 315CE and the 6th century at the order of a Christian emperor named Theodosius

(408-450). In 782 CE, Emperor Charlemagne ordered the beheading of 4500 Saxons when they refused to convert to Christianity. During the crusades (1095-1291), millions of nonbelievers were slaughtered. From the beginning of Christianity until 1484, several thousand witches were burned at the stake or hung. During the years of Spanish conquistadores and Columbus's journey to the Americas, millions of natives were killed in the name of Christianity (1500–1900). The horrors of the Spanish inquisition in 1478 led to the murder of thousands of Jews and Muslims. Millions of Jews were massacred by Hitler, a Catholic, during World War II. Such are the paradoxes of religion—"Be cruel and kill to be kind and survive" (Paradox Definition and meaning, www.dictionary.com).

CHAPTER 10

What Lies Ahead In The Treatment Of Violent And Deviant Behavior, One Hundred Years From Today?

Epigenetics, Genetic Manipulation And Nanotechnology

"The Church angrily denounced the introduction of medicines, antibiotics, anesthesia, surgery, blood transfusions, birth control, in vitro fertilization and most forms of pain killers. Supposedly, these scientific tools interfered with nature and were therefore against God's will. Today, the Church is fighting stem-cell research, cloning technology and genetic engineering" **– David Mills –author of *Atheist Universe: The Thinking Person's Answer to Christian Fundamentalism***

"The advance of genetic engineering makes it quite conceivable that we will begin to design our own evolutionary progress" **– Isaac Asimov (1920-1992), American writer and professor of biochemistry**

"It should soon be possible dramatically to increase the intelligence and life span of a few individuals. They and their offspring could become a master race. Evolution pays no regards to social justice. It was not fair on Neanderthals they were replaced by modern humans" **– Stephen Hawking**

"Every time you understand something, religion becomes less likely. Only with the discovery of the double helix and the ensuing genetic revolution have we had grounds for thinking that the powers held traditionally to be the exclusive property of the gods might one day be ours…" **– James D Watson – American molecular biologist, geneticist, and zoologist**

While religion joyously relishes and celebrates the events that occurred thousands of years ago and continues to propagate its belief system, science continues its never-ending quest to explore and explain the unknowns and take a close look at the minute structures that constitute the entire human body. Vaccines have become available to prevent deadly microbial infections. Humans have reached the moon and Mars and explored distant planets in the solar system. Water was found under the surface of the red planet. In 1996, a sheep named Dolly was cloned. In 2001, the first artificial heart that powers itself was created by Massachusetts-based AbioMed. In 2003, geneticists successfully sequenced the entire human genome. Approximately 23,000 genes were sequenced that shed light on many aspects of our lives, including treatment of various diseases, evolution, cloning, and gene therapy. Manipulation of the genetic makeup of plants is now common. Sequencing of DNA fragments was pioneered by and developed independently by Walter Gilbert and Frederick Sanger, who won Nobel prizes in 1980 for their work. In 2007, the ability of stem cells to transform themselves and become any type of cell was exploited to grow organs like kidney, lung, heart, and brain. In 2012, a collaborative effort by researchers at Harvard University and the University of California at Berkeley led to gene-editing technology that can change the way physicians treat infectious disease by cutting out pieces of harmful DNA. Mobile phone technology, driverless cars, and electric cars are here to stay, and continue to improve and advance as we speak. Recently, a $10 billion James Webb telescope captured stunning images of several galaxies several million light years away. A NASA spaceship launched on November 23, 2021 in an experiment to deflect an asteroid hit its target on September 26, 2022. Although the asteroid was not actually a threat, this feat demonstrated mans' ability to stop or deflect an incoming celestial object from colliding with the Earth.

The microscopic materials that hold the key to the origin and propagation of life are located inside the nucleus of a cell, and inside the nucleus are rod-shaped structures called chromosomes. The human genome is the complete set of full DNA content assembled and contained in 46 chromosomes in 23 pairs: 22 autosomes and a pair of sex chromosomes, X and Y. The autosomes determine the traits of the individual and the sex chromosomes determine the gender of the individual. Each chromosome contains deoxyribonucleic acid or DNA, that forms the genes—the basis of heredity. Each human chromosome contains approximately 20,000–25,000 genes.

The nucleic acids DNA and RNA (ribonucleic acid) are composed of three types of units: a five-carbon sugar (deoxyribose in DNA and ribose in RNA), a nitrogen-containing base (purines and pyrimidines), and phosphate. DNA has two purine bases (adenine and guanine) and two pyrimidines (thymine and cytosine). The DNA molecule, or the "Watson-Crick double helix," carries the biochemical basis of heredity. The helix has polynucleotide chains held together by hydrogen bonds between pairs of bases—adenine (A) paired with thymine (T,) and guanine (G) paired with cytosine (C). Genetic information is stored in the DNA molecule by means of a code with an infinite number of variations. Vital to the understanding of the mechanisms of epigenetics is knowing the chemical constituents of the chromosomes and the chromatin structures that are wrapped around histone proteins, as discussed later in this chapter.

Any discussion of DNA must include mitochondrial DNA. The genetic materials are located in the mitochondria and in the nucleus of eukaryotic cells. They contain genes essential for the synthesis of adenosine triphosphate, the cell's main source of energy. Mitochondrial DNA is inherited exclusively via the maternal line. Organs affected by mitochondrial disorders include the brain, muscles, nerves, eyes, ears, heart, liver, and kidneys, organs that are also affected by various medical conditions including connective tissue and autoimmune diseases, sarcoidosis, and infectious diseases.

The DNA helix resembles the Sumerian double helix snake god, the Caduceus, and the Rod of Asclepius. Asclepius is the god of medicine in Greek mythology. The rod has a single snake without wings, while the Caduceus is a winged staff with two snakes wrapped around the rod. They are both used as symbols of medicine. Is it possible that the double helix snake god is a representation of the DNA helix that was carved in stone by the Sumerians (or by those gods who descended from the sky) for modern humans to decipher?

The union between the spermatozoon (male cell) and the ovum (female cell) is the beginning of a complex series of cellular proliferation, migration, exchange, and transfer of genetic materials between a man and a woman. Soon, three germ cell layers—ectoderm, mesoderm, and endoderm—are formed, from which various organs are derived. The endoderm gives rise to the respiratory tract, the urinary bladder, the thyroid and parathyroid, the liver and pancreas, tonsils, the thymus gland, and the epithelia of the tympanic membrane. The mesoderm gives rise to striated and nonstriated muscles, cartilage and bone, connective tissues, the dura, the parietal peritoneum and pleura, the endocardium and myocardium, blood and lymphatic vessels, the gonads, the spleen, and the adrenal glands. The brain and spinal cord, skin, the sensory epithelia of the eyes, ears and nose, the mammary glands, pituitary gland, tooth enamel, sinuses, and oral cavities are derived from the ectoderm. Just like any other organs, the brain, which represents the central nervous system, can be affected by various diseases, with manifestations that depend on the specific parts affected.

When the brain is damaged by trauma, malignant tumor, infection, or degenerative conditions, such as Alzheimer disease, Huntington's disease, prion disorders, and various dementias, a person suffering from any of these diseases is treated with sympathy and compassion. A person suffering from psychoses, such as schizophrenia and major depressive disorders, is also treated with understanding and some degree of sympathy. On the other hand, a person with a personality disorder (narcissistic, borderline personality, obsessive compulsive, anti-social, paranoid, or schizoid behavior), sexual attraction to minors (pedophilia), or sexual aggression is treated with indifference, disdain, and hatred by the general public. With a proper understanding of neuroscience, homosexuality—which is condemned by some religious groups—is now accepted as a standard norm in this modern-day society; this is a step forward in the right direction. Unfortunately, but realistically, these aberrant behaviors will always be judged based on spiritual and religious laws, and not by the preponderance of anatomical, physiological, and chemical abnormalities demonstrated in the brains of these people. At this time, no matter how science treats this issue, sexual predators and murderers will always be ostracized and condemned by religious groups and punished by the current legal system.

At the level of molecular genetics, all body organs, including the brain, are subject to some defect in cellular organization, which makes them susceptible to acquiring certain diseases—or the acquisition of rogue neural connections in the case of the limbic system. Assessment of pharmacological treatments (antiandrogens, luteinizing hormone-release hormone antagonists, and serotonergics) for aberrant behavior, particularly pedophilia, has been difficult to extrapolate, and these treatments do not decrease the recidivism rate. The recent state of knowledge indicates that cognitive-behavioral psychotherapy is the method of choice. Unfortunately, it is not a cure, and the threat of relapse is always present. Currently, no biomarkers are available to serve as diagnostic tools to determine the proclivity to develop pedophilia and other perverted behaviors. The complexity and variability of pre- and perinatal factors add to the difficulty in searching for biomarkers.

Can genetic manipulation prevent rogue behavior from overtly manifesting itself after birth, but before that person harboring the defective genes becomes a menace to society? A specific gene locus in a particular chromosome that puts an individual at risk for developing certain behavioral disorders has yet to be identified. Recent genetic investigations, however, have demonstrated several genes (called NRXN1, HTR2A, CTTNBP2, and REEP3) associated with OCD, a complex disorder involving both genetic and environmental factors. In addition, genome-wide linkage analysis has shown a suggestive linkage on the short arm of chromosome 1 in OCD, as well as major depressive disorder. Evidence for a linkage was also found on chromosomes 1, 4, 9, and 18, with the highest linkage on the short arm of chromosome 9, in borderline personality disorders. Variations in a gene called CACNA1C that codes for cellular machinery that regulates calcium influx into neurons has been associated with bipolar disorder, schizophrenia, and major depression. The CACNB2 gene, and certain regions in chromosomes 3 and 10, have also been found to be linked in these disorders, as well as autism. Reports of chromosomal aberrations in bipolar disorder have been demonstrated but the specific gene has yet to be identified. Regions of interest include the short arm of chromosome 4 (4p16), the long arm of chromosome 12 (12q23-q24),the long arm of chromosome 21 (21q22), and the long arm of the X chromosome (Xq24-q26). To date, several genes on chromosome 6 that regulate immune function have emerged as a chromosomal abnormality associated with a risk of schizophrenia. A rare deletion on chromosome 16 is more common among schizophrenics than in healthy controls. In a large study, rare deletions in chromosomes 1, 15, and 22 were found among 5,000 schizophrenics but not in 41,000 controls.

An emerging and innovative technique known as epigenetic engineering (or editing) may become a game changer. Epigenetics (prefix "epi-"means "above" or "upon") is the study of how behaviors and the environment can cause changes that affect the activities of the genes (phenotype) without altering the DNA sequence (genotype). These changes are vital to normal biological functioning, and they affect the natural cycles of cellular death, renewal, and replacement, and aging. Lifestyle and behavioral factors, such as diet, sleep, exercise, smoking, and alcohol; environmental factors, such as toxins, stress and trauma; and place of residence can affect and alter the composition and location of the chemical groups that bind to DNA. In recent years, research on epigenetics has been extended to nonhuman primates and to humans. Early life experiences impact the future of the personality development of the young. Animal models provide evidence that early-life adversarial relationships can produce long-lasting epigenetic changes in the brain, particularly in the limbic system. Maternal licking in rodents, a form of pleasant grooming behavior similar to caressing human babies, activates all regions in the limbic system, resulting in calming effect, trust, and assurance. By contrast, babies and children deprived of parental nurturing, and those subjected to abuse, will have difficulty adjusting to future daily life experiences, such as stress and adversarial challenges. In essence, epigenetic mechanisms impact brain development and are nature's way to enable the young to adapt to a specific social environment. This means that the young, when living in a harsh environment, will learn how to be defensive and vigilant and to mistrust people. By contrast, a child who grows up in a friendly environment with nurturing adults will develop emotional stability, empathy, and cognitive flexibility.

Epigenetic changes can be passed down to future generations. These changes can even occur in plants, fungi, and invertebrates. An example of how the environment can affect epigenetics is the Dutch famine of 1944–1945. Studies have shown that children born during that period have a higher rate of coronary artery disease and obesity because their mothers were exposed to famine. The opposite was observed in children not exposed to famine.

Epigenetics is now being applied in several medical fields, particularly oncology, regenerative medicine, infectious diseases, and neuropsychiatry. The disruption of epigenetic processes is now well established to lead to altered gene function and malignant transformation of normal cells. Although this line of research is still in an early stage of development, it greatly improves our understanding of neuronal plasticity, and it may eventually lead to innovative and fundamentally effective therapy for various medical conditions. It is a promising strategy in cancer therapy, because epigenetic aberrations are reversible. The field of oncology now uses chemical, and biologic agents to enable transformed cells to function in a normal way. The FDA has approved a number of drugs that target epigenetic regulation to treat various malignancies, such as myelodysplastic syndrome, multiple myeloma, and T-cell lymphoma. Epigenetic mechanisms, which are intrinsically reversible and dynamic in the regulation of chromatic structure, can regulate the determination of stem and progenitor cell fates. The sophisticated ability of some microbials to evade the action of antibiotics and circumvent the body's immune system can be neutralized by modifying the epigenetic changes in histone acetylation in the DNA.

Epigenetic mechanisms are involved in the development of the central nervous system and play a major role in the pathophysiology of various psychiatric disorders, such as bipolar disorder, depression, and schizophrenia. Recent epigenetic research supports the idea that adverse psychosocial experiences are associated with psychiatric disorders, such as schizophrenia, anxiety, depression, and substance addiction, while positive epigenetic associations have been observed with cognitive and behavioral therapy, diet, and exercise.

What are the mechanisms involved in epigenetics? Understanding the intricacies of the long strands of DNA composition and the arrangement of molecules inside the nuclei is vital. Although humans are born with a set of genes made from DNA (the genome), epigenetics focuses on how the traits are expressed through various modifications of chemicals around or outside the genome (the "epigenome"). While genetic changes refer to the production of proteins upon instructions from the DNA, epigenetic changes affect gene expression by switching genes "on" and "off." These actions are influenced by behavior and environmental elements. The epigenome is the target point of epigenetics, where chemical actions are located outside the genome. The opening and closing of the chromatin wrapped around the histone proteins will determine the transcription and translation of protein through the action of RNA (ribonucleic acid) and the polymerase enzyme. RNA has several forms, each with its own function (messenger RNA, transfer RNA, microRNA, and non-coding RNA). They all mediate the transfer of the language of the DNA sequence that leads to the formation of proteins.

Epigenetic changes affect gene expression in different ways. Frequently investigated epigenetic mechanisms for changes in chromatin structure are DNA methylation, histone modification, and microRNA (Figure 4). Blood is the usual peripheral tissue for the study DNA methylation. Samples from umbilical tissues are used to assay changes in chromatin structure. Cancer cells are used in oncology research and therapy. In animal studies, brain tissues are studied directly. An important point to note is that the methylation pattern in the blood does not necessarily or accurately reflect the pattern in the brain. However, recent studies have shown that regions in the human genome for some profiled organs, such as thyroid, heart, and brain tissue, were associated with genes implicated in a broad range of phenotypes and diseases. In essence, DNA methylation in one tissue will correlate with gene expression in another tissue. Given the appropriate clinical history and symptomatology in an individual with a certain behavioral problem, this finding supports the use of peripheral tissue like blood to assess gene methylation. Notably, these epigenetic mechanisms, particularly methylation, are highest in newborns and lowest in the very elderly. Epigenetics is therefore an ongoing process that begins even before birth.

DNA methylation is the most frequently studied epigenetic modification. It involves binding of a methyl group (CH_3) to the cytosine base of DNA, catalyzed by the enzyme DNA methyltransferase. This resulting chemical group can be demethylated, creating the "off" (methylation) and "on" (demethylation) process, depending on various environmental factors, medical conditions, aging, diet, and stress. This process regulates gene expression by turning off the gene function and stabilizing cell differentiation, as in the transformation of normal cells into malignant forms. A link between poor diet, epigenetics, and DNA methylation has been established, and is manifested clinically as an increased risk of behavioral problems and autism. The process has also been associated with increased activity of the hypothalamic, pituitary-adrenal axis resulting in anxiety, depression, and increased levels of cortisol in newborns of depressed mothers.

The other epigenetic process is called histone modification. Histone proteins act to package DNA tightly to form the chromosomal structure inside the nucleus. This process of modification involves various enzymatic reactions that include phosphorylation, methylation, acetylation, ubiquitylation, and sumoylation. SUMO proteins are small ubiquitin-like modifier proteins that belong to a family of small proteins that covalently attach to and detach from other proteins to modify their functions. The product of these reactions is post-translational modification to histone proteins, which alters the chromatin structure. When histones become loosely packed, more DNA is exposed, enabling the reactions to take place easily so the gene is turned "on". These chemical groups can be removed to retighten the histones ("off"). Elucidation of histone modification patterns has important implications for stem cell and cancer research and provides targets for combating tumor cell proliferation, leading to new diagnostic and therapeutic approaches in various medical disorders, such as cancer.

Beyond the level of DNA methylation (involved in the cellular control of gene expression and aberrant hypermethylation) and histone modification (involved in the control of the accessibility of chromatin and transcriptional activities inside the cell) is another epigenetic mechanism that is less well understood. It involves microRNAs (miRNAs), small non-coding RNA (ncRNA) molecules that control posttranscriptional gene expression. Recently, the expression of miRNAs has been linked to cancer development. Around 98% of the genome does not code for proteins, making miRNAs significant participants in gene expression, as they can attach to coding RNA and recruit proteins to modify histones to turn the genes "on" and "off." The ncRNAs have also been found to suppress and activate gene expression at the levels of transcription and translation. Studies have shown that circulating miRNAs are involved in the pathogenesis, diagnosis, and prognosis of depression and can be used as potential biomarkers for this condition. Some researchers have discovered that miRNAs may mediate anxiety-like symptoms.

There is every reason to believe that epigenetics has a role in religious indoctrination. It is well known that religion involves a sophisticated system of belief inculcated in the limbic system of innocent children. Physical and social environmental factors, childhood training within the family circle, and nurturing can alter gene expression and these changes can be passed down from one generation to another without altering the basic genome of a child. A set of identical twins, raised by two parents, one a Christian and the other a Muslim, will develop contrasting religious practices as they grow up. A child raised by atheist parents and trained to recognize right from wrong without invoking a supernatural being will likely wonder why his Christian and Muslim friends go to a place of worship every week. It is clear that epigenetic influence can be expressed as variations in personality and individuality. It should be noted, however, that the basic genome may still play a role in the individual's susceptibility and resistance to certain disease processes, such as infection, cancer, and diabetes.

Can epigenetics offer solutions to prevent school shootings? The optimistic answer is yes. In general, deaths from firearms comprise only a small proportion of childhood deaths, but mass killings in schools are a serious public concern. Many mass shootings originate from various factors, such as history of parental abuse, ineffective parenting, mental illness, school bullying, drugs, easy access to firearms, and availability of violent video games and movies. A combination of these factors may lead to feelings of rejection, isolation, envy, and rebellion, and motivate the youth to act violently in revenge. If epigenetics can alter gene expression and groom children to develop attitudes and behaviors of practical value in the society where they live and to obtain social usefulness and maximum individual development, it makes sense that all these factors can be controlled to prevent these tragedies from happening. Although optimistically simplistic, society has to start doing something and take advantage of what science, not prayers, can offer.

The moral condemnation of homosexuality is well known and is recorded in the Bible. Homosexuals have been ridiculed, stigmatized, and ostracized, even in modern society. Not too long ago, they were blamed for the spread of the human immunodeficiency virus. In the past, they suffered from gruesome punishments—thrown from high buildings or stoned to death—for their behavior. In addition to several neuroanatomical and neurophysiological findings discovered in the brain of homosexuals (Chapter 3), the science of epigenetics has recently provided a plausible explanation for the development of homosexuality. It is well established that fetal androgen signaling may be linked to sexual development. While humans are born with a basic DNA sequence, the development of future phenotypic changes is influenced by gene expression modulated by several factors, such as environment, stress, family upbringing, and hormones. It is reasonable to hypothesize that homosexuality is acquired through epigenetic transformation and not by the presence of a "gay" gene per se. Studies have shown that the genes of identical twins, although genomically identical, may not be exactly identical, and can be expressed differently in subsequent years after birth. This has been shown among identical twins, in which one twin is homosexual whereas the other is not and only has 20-50% chance of being homosexual. Other studies have shown that sexual orientation is more concordant in monozygotic twins than in dizygotic twins. Another study on monozygotic twin pairs, however, showed no support for the epigenetic hypothesis. Therefore, at this time, the jury is still out, and it remains speculative that sexual orientation is linked to epigenetic mechanisms or to androgen signaling. Be that as it may, numerous neuroanatomical findings, as discussed in Chapter 3, have been associated with homosexuality.

Is there a relationship between epigenetics and quantum mechanics (QM)? Is it possible that changes in gene expression are mediated by QM—a fundamental theory in physics that provides a description of the physical properties of everything in nature at the atomic and subatomic level? Quantum phenomena are present all around and are acting at every scale. The science of QM may even reveal how everything in the universe is interconnected, and it has the potential to transform human views of gravity and its relation to space and time. QM has shown that matter and energy are in the form of discrete packets or "quanta," and, in the case of light, energy is delivered in quanta that consist of "photons." Given the fact that everything in the universe is interconnected, could it be that the actions of various neurotransmitters located and stored in the neuronal synapses in the limbic system and brainstem are driven by QM? The Dalai Lama remarked, "Within every atom, you can find part of the stardust that comes from the very beginning of the universe. We're all connected and form part of the same essence. Understanding this connection can help us understand the importance of being good. That's because you do reverberate in the universe and comes back to you."

At the "macro" level, everything in the universe that moves is demonstrable visually. The moons revolve around planets, which, in turn, revolve around stars. Billions of stars comprise a galaxy, and along with other galaxies, they constitute the universe . The galaxies are held together by a powerful but yet to be seen force that astrophysicists call "dark matter." At the "micro" level, a speck of dust in a planet is composed of several quadrillion atoms. An atom is the building block of matter. It consists of 3 subatomic particles known as protons, neutrons, and electrons. The protons and neutrons form the nucleus of the atom around which are electron shells that contain electrons that orbit the nucleus at high speed.

Parallel to the emergence and development of epigenetics, and perhaps soon converging together in the field of medicine is nanotechnology, the study and application of extremely small particles that are used across several scientific fields, such as chemistry, biology, physics, and engineering. It is science, engineering, and technology conducted at the nanoscale, which is about 1 to 10 nanometers or a billionth of a meter. One nanometer is about the size of six bonded carbon atoms. Comparatively, approximately 40,000 nanometers are equivalent to the width of a human hair. Another way to visualize and measure a nanometer is to look at the size of a red blood cell, which is approximately 7000 nm in diameter, while a white blood cell diameter is 10,000 nm, a virus is 100 nm, and a hydrogen atom is 0.1 nm. Nanoparticles range from 1–100nm. The concept of nanoscience was first introduced during a lecture given by Richard Feynman at an American Physical Society Meeting at the California Institute of Technology in 1959, in which he discussed a process by which scientists would be able to manipulate and control atoms and molecules. A decade later, in 1974, Professor Norio Taniguchi at the University of Tokyo coined the term "nano-technology." Another decade later, in 1986, Foresight Nanotech Institute founder K. Eric Drexler introduced the term "molecular nanotechnology."

There are different types of nanoparticles, and they are classified according to size, morphology, and physical and chemical properties. They are natural or man-made, and organic or inorganic. Some are carbon-based, while others are made of ceramic, metal, and semiconductor materials. Polymers and lipid nanoparticles are currently being studied as delivery systems for nucleic acids used in gene therapy.

Nanotechnology has the potential to change everything in the practice of medicine. It is being studied in the diagnosis of atherosclerosis, development of gene sequencing, delivery of medications directly to cancer cells, repair of spinal injuries, refinement of vaccine delivery, and creation of crystal mineral structures for dental restoration. A few decades from today, it will be used routinely in the treatment of various psychiatric disorders. Pharmacotherapy for depression, although effective in most situations, is not without serious side effects. The efficacy wanes over time. Tragic paradoxical reactions like suicides have been reported to occur. Perfection of nanotechnology can deliver drugs selectively to regulate serotonergic and dopaminergic neurons and synapses. It has the potential to regulate epigenetic mechanisms, such as DNA methylation, histone protein modification, and miRNAs.

Pharmacology and nanotechnology have begun to intersect in the treatment of pain syndromes. Conventionally, when drugs are delivered to the site of a pain generator, unwanted reactions may potentially occur, not to mention the adverse effects on other organs. The use of nanoparticles to deliver drug molecules specifically to the source of pain is an innovative way to circumvent adverse reactions. Similarly, delivery of psychopharmacologic drugs to the limbic system can be accomplished with precision to treat major psychoses and personality disorders. However, obstacles need to be overcome, including allergic and autoimmune reactions, long-term side effects, potential toxicities, the expense of the procedure, and the establishment of criteria and proper patient selection. Acute and long-term side effects have yet to be fully assessed in laboratory animals. The carcinogenic potential of the nanoparticles, as well as adverse effects, including premature aging, neurological dysfunction, facilitation of cardiovascular atherosclerosis, and effects on other organs, have potentially serious outcomes.

Epigenetic mechanisms

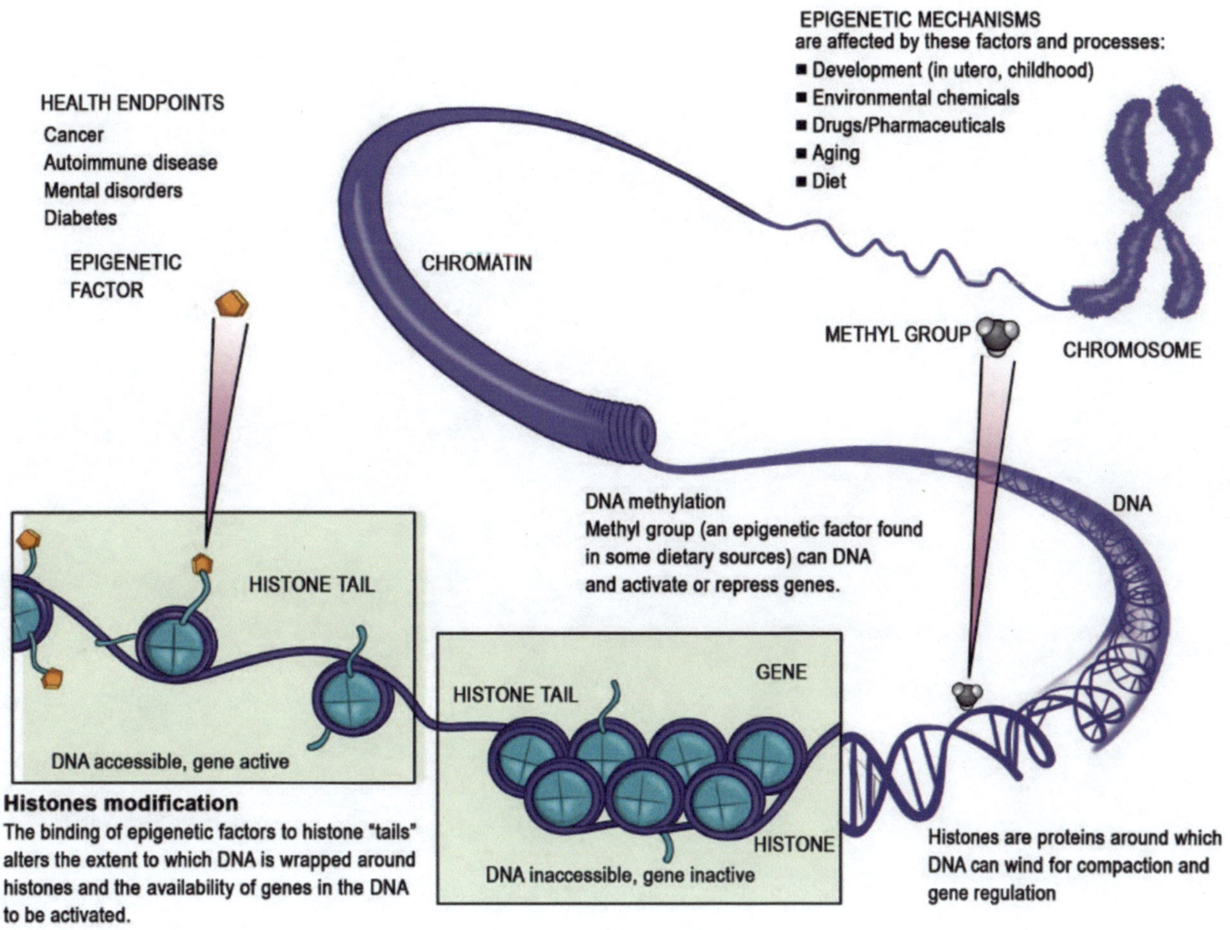

Diagram of the EPIGENOMICS – Modified from the original scientific illustration obtained from the National Institutes of Health, Office of Strategic Coordination – The Common Fund.

Shown are the processes of methylation and histone modification. Methylation works by adding a chemical group, Methyl (CH_3), to DNA. DNA surrounds and wraps around highly basic proteins called histones that function to compress DNA within the nucleus to form the chromatin, which regulates gene transcription. Beyond the level of methylation and histone modification is called microRNAs, a type of small non-coding RNA molecules that control posttranscript gene expression. Coding RNA is used to make proteins. Attachment of non-coding RNA to coding RNA helps regulate gene expression and recruitment of proteins which is essential to modify histones.

CHAPTER 11

Reflections And Realities

Practical And Thought-Provoking Questions

"They told me to use the brain God gave me. I did. Now I am an atheist. Ironic, isn't it?" – **atheist saying (www.geckoandfly.com)**

"Religious dogma creates a perfect fertilizer for the weed of hypocrisy" – **Steve Maraboli**

"The most important thing is to never stop questioning" – **Albert Einstein**

"Study the science of art. Study the art of science. Develop your senses—especially learn how to see. Realize that everything connects to everything else" – **Leonardo da Vinci (1452-1519), Italian Renaissance polymath, scientist, engineer, and painter**

If the sixth commandment is to be followed, then the destiny of a person living in a congested urban city who grew up in a one-parent family in a neighborhood riddled with drugs, crime, and prostitution, who viciously killed somebody on the street while trying to defend himself or while trying to rob an innocent person on the street, is likely hell. If a man with a recent history of hypersexuality rapes a woman and later dies of an undiagnosed brain tumor that had destroyed his orbitofrontal cortex, will his soul go to hell? The Bible disapproves of homosexuality, so will the soul of a homosexual person go to hell? If a person who grew up in a family whose members are corrupt politicians who have committed graft and corruption several times, will his or her soul go to hell if that person commits the same misdeeds? If a priest, who after 8 years of studying in the seminary and making a pledge to serve the community and God, was found later to be a pedophile, will his soul go to hell or heaven? If a person does not (and refuses to) believe in God and never attends religious rites but never commits a crime, and is simply a good person, will that person's soul go to hell or heaven upon death? If a person is trained by parents and clergy to hate and kill followers of another religion, where will that person's soul go? If the soul goes to hell, why will that person be blamed for these actions? If a habitual criminal becomes brain-dead following a serious accident and his family members decided to donate his organs to a dying but very nice religious person, who later dies after several years of being supported by the organs from that criminal, where will the religious soul go? Will half of the soul (the half without those organs) go to heaven, and the other half (with those organs) to hell? These are practical questions about sinful acts that believers and their Bible ought to be able to answer without putting an "evasive spin" on the issues.

Science has demonstrated the higher centers in the brain that control and regulate most of our actions across human history, and people have found ways to get along well. Aggression is a term for behavior intended to cause harm to others and is manifested as responses ranging from verbal anger and use of foul language to vicious physical attacks. It evolved as a protective adaptation to deal with competition, and it is basically influenced by complex interactions among genes, neural circuitry, and the environment. The center for aggressive behavior resides in an area located in the ventral and medial hypothalamus—the area that, when affected by adverse side effects of certain medications, social threats, or environmental circumstances, can cause an individual to become violent.

Hypersexuality or compulsive sexual behavior is an excessive preoccupation with sexual fantasies, urges, or behaviors that are difficult to control. It can have a negative effect on mental health. Anatomical differences are largely due to sex hormones. Females have a greater volume in the prefrontal cortex, orbitofrontal cortex, superior temporal cortex, lateral parietal cortex, and insula. Males, on average, have greater volume in the ventral temporal and occipital regions. Regions with relatively high expression of sex-chromosome genes tend to have greater cortical volume in males than in females. In pathological situations, hypersexuality has been reported to occur in some people with Alzheimer's dementia, frontotemporal dementia, Parkinson's Disease, autism, various brain injuries, attention deficit hyperactivity disorder, and partial complex seizures. Obviously, these conditions are causally related to abnormal neuronal circuitry that leads to disruption and imbalance of behavior-mediating neurotransmitters, such as serotonin, norepinephrine, and dopamine. Per se, sexual aggression is considered a sin. Where will the souls of those people with the aforementioned conditions go? Are they responsible for their actions? What does the Bible say? The answer is "Nothing," because everything in the Bible is about mind control, not science.

Some patients with Tourette's syndrome, a neurodevelopmental disorder, have involuntary utterances of obscenities and profanities, along with uncontrollable motor tics. Outbursts of derogatory and racial remarks may also occur. Obscenities and profanities are considered verbal forms of aggression and sinful acts by the Bible. Does the soul of a person with Tourette's syndrome go to hell?

All believers and religious people are quick to attribute sins as acts against divine law, and they have the mindset that every human action, good or bad, is spiritually mediated, while totally ignoring the biological and organic aspect of an action. It is quite difficult to understand that people with abnormal neuronal circuitry and imbalances in their neurotransmitters due to various neurological disorders, for no fault of their own, will be sent down to hell. These are people created by the almighty God, but why will God punish the objects of his own creation?

Epigenetic mechanisms and nanotechnology are here to stay and will likely play a major role in grooming the behavior and daily activities of humans from all walks of life 50 to 100 years from today. Anxiety, depression, various personality disorders, infectious diseases, cancer, neurodegenerative disorders, metabolic disorders, and various inherited diseases may become things of the past. Drug delivery to kill cancer cells can be done with precision without inducing adverse side effects on other organs. Rewiring the aberrant neural connections and correcting the imbalances in various neurotransmitters in psychoses, such as major depression and schizophrenia, using nanotechnology may no longer be considered science fiction. Regenerative medicine (stem cell implants and gene therapy) will be perfected soon. Quantum mechanics are looming on the horizon.

What about religious indoctrination? Religion, very much like politics, divides, deludes, and ostracizes people. It promotes hatred and bigotry. Millions of people all over the world have died at the hands of Christian explorers spreading the religion of Christianity. Followers of major religions have waged war against each other. The everlasting reward of going to heaven and fear of eternal damnation in hell are the powerful, but unfortunate, central themes of indoctrination. Reports of apparitions, dramatizations of religious events by Hollywood movies, and reports of miracles are spiritual and inspirational wonders for believers but ridiculously nonsensical for freethinkers and nonbelievers. If the mind can be groomed and re-wired by epigenetic mechanisms and nanotechnology—which is happening as we speak—the same processes may also be applied to those religious people who wish to change the way they live or those who wish to escape from the powerful grip of religion and realize that prayers do not really work.

Obviously, seeing the future is not possible unless the fictional time machine becomes a reality. Be that as it may, what will happen to a society that is free of crime, free of so-called sinful acts, free not to practice any religion, and free to eliminate the unfounded belief in a never-been-seen supernatural deity? Are inhabitants of the planet Earth better off with the status quo and letting faith dictate their lives? Faith, which is based on spiritual apprehension rather than proof, promotes weakness and helplessness among humans as it stems from fear of eternal punishment—fear inculcated into the mind of the innocent children before they reach the age of reason. Moreover, religion has always been the source of conflicts, hatred, and social divisions in this world. As it stands right now, people want to live peacefully without fear of intimidation and threat, and they strive to eliminate these from their lives.

"This would be the best of all worlds if there were no religion in it" – John Adams (1735-1826), 2nd President of the US, statesman, lawyer, diplomat, writer, and founding father

Checks and balances and "ecology" in animal society have been the norms for thousands of years. The saying goes that "for every action, there is an equal and opposite reaction." For an animal to exist, both pleasant and noxious stimuli must exist at the same time for proper adaptation in the environment in which it lives. Microbials exist and multiply by feeding on tissue substrates in the animal body, while the latter develops a defense system by producing white blood cells and antibodies to combat the former. Carbon dioxide, along with water and sunlight, are needed by plants for photosynthesis, the by-products of which are oxygen molecules needed by animals to maintain cardiac and pulmonary functions and help metabolize the foods they eat. One of the by-products of this metabolism is carbon dioxide molecules, released into the environment for re-consumption by plants—and so the endless cycling and recycling of life go on and on.

One would wonder where humans are heading to, while relentless and countless accomplishments by science continue to move on nonstop. If humans use their senses rationally and avoid nuclear war, the unknowns in this universe will soon be revealed—without the help of prayers. People will not only be interested in the future but will also be intrigued to know what exactly happened in the past that led to the development of religion and a supernatural deity.

Of course, it is all about a belief system. Followers are forbidden to ask what, why, when, and how, or risk condemnation and even a death sentence. So many events described in the Bible and ancient writings need further scrutiny. For example, how was it possible, realistically, to impregnate the Virgin Mary without sexual intercourse? Was she impregnated via in vitro fertilization by advanced or extraterrestrial beings in the past? Was she really a virgin, and did she remain a virgin following birth of Jesus Christ? How was it possible to part the Red Sea while the Jewish people were trying to escape from Egyptian persecution? Jesus suffered and died for the so-called sins of mankind. But how is sin defined in a person with abnormal neural fabric in the limbic lobe or someone who harbors a brain tumor or neurodegenerative disorders who becomes violent while a neurological disease is progressing?

There are 15 million Jews in the world, and not all of them believe that Jesus is the son of God or the messiah. Christians believe the opposite. Islam considers Jesus a prophet but neither God nor a son of God. It condemns homosexuality. Why did the ground shake and why thunder and lightning (and loud "trumpets") on Mount Sinai when Moses received the Ten Commandments? What is the true identity of Jesus Christ? What led the ancients to consider him a son of God? If he was reincarnated following his death on the cross, why have modern humans not seen him walking around urban cities combatting crimes? Who created the Neanderthals and *Homo sapiens*, who existed long before Adam and Eve were supposedly created by God. Who created the Sumerians, an advanced civilization in Mesopotamia that existed between 6000–11,000 BC? Adam and Eve are portrayed as white Caucasians. The Christians claim all humans originated from that couple. Does this mean that black Africans, American Indians, Philippine negritos, Australian aborigines, and Japanese and Chinese people originated from Adam and Eve? These are important and practical questions, but believers would rather avoid discussing them because they do not have answers.

Also, regarding pedophiles (including clergy members who abuse minors), psychotics or non-psychotics who exhibit hypersexuality or hyperreligiosity, people with frequent out-of-body experiences, serial killers, religious people who experience recurrent bouts of illusory after-images (palinopsia) and repetitive perception of sound after physical noise has disappeared (palinacousis), and previously healthy people who subacutely develop depression and hallucinations—should these people undergo routine neurological evaluation and neurodiagnostic examination to look for brain tumors, epilepsy, unusual infection, autoimmune disease, and/or degenerative disorders? How many people suffered from those disorders in ancient times and were mistakenly judged to be possessed by demons and then burned at the stake or stoned to death? The past is the bridge to the future, and the future will provide the bridge for those believers to allow them to understand the real world outside their steel cage of religion.

> *"Religions are all alike—founded upon fables and mythologies."* – **Thomas Jefferson (1743-1826), founding father and 3rd President of the U.S., statesman, lawyer, diplomat, architect, philosopher**
>
> *"Just because you believe in something does not mean it is true."* – **Albert Einstein**
>
> *"The key to the future lies hidden in the past."* – **Erich Von Daniken – author of *Chariots of the Gods* and several books on ancient gods and extraterrestrial visitations**

The fate of humanity is speculative. Its future is largely a function of our future society and government, but it will continue to know no bounds as they continue to evolve. If humanity is heading to the future without being interrupted by nuclear war, is it likely that a perfect world society will emerge? How will a perfect society be defined? What are the ramifications of such a society? Most diseases will likely be controlled or prevented, and aging will be slowed down, thereby increasing the human lifespan. This increase will inevitably occur as humans prepare for interstellar journeys to reach other habitable solar systems, since our sun will continue to age and run out of the hydrogen fuel in its core. It will soon burn the helium layer, expand, become a red giant, and engulf the inner planets—Mercury, Venus, and Earth—and possibly Mars and the gaseous planets. It will then shrink and become a white dwarf.

In this world, the presence of various racial ideologies, social practices, and various religions (there are approximately 4000 in this world), along with the instinctive protection of territorial boundaries and the never ending immiscibility of religion and science, will always generate mistrust, malice, deception, cheating, greed, covetousness, insolence, religious wars, envy, libel, slander, malfeasance among government officials, back-stabbings, and intimidations. Although epigenetic mechanisms and nanotechnology can potentially rectify the aberrant neural pathways responsible for the generation of various neuropsychiatric disorders, possibly within the next one hundred years, this approach cannot be logistically undertaken on a global scale at the present time. As science continues to advance, future generations of believers will finally come to their senses and realize that diseases can only be treated by science and that natural disasters and celestial cataclysms cannot be prevented by prayers and miracles. People will realize that the claims of miraculous improvement and survival of certain incurable medical disorders as a result of prayers were more likely a result of misdiagnosis. Sinful acts forbidden by the Ten Commandments will persist for as long as the neurotransmitter activities are dysregulated. People with bad genes and abnormal neural connections in their limbic system who happen to live in crime-infested urban cities will continue to get involved in violent crimes, pornography, and crimes against the weaker sex. Those who tenaciously believe in the existence of the soul and out-of-body experiences (or near-death experiences) will soon be convinced that they have been misinformed and hoodwinked by religious indoctrination.

In the U.S., the decline of Christianity continues at a rapid pace as young adults lose faith in religion. The belief system and faith will soon be replaced by belief in and reliance on the medical and technological accomplishments of science. The millions of people who died during the COVID pandemic and natural disasters were not saved by prayers. Earthquakes, hurricanes, tornadoes, floods, volcanic eruptions, microbial pandemics, and collision with celestial objects will continue to kill thousands and millions of people, including believers and nonbelievers alike. Nations ruled by dictators and tyrants will continue to intimidate other nations and be a menace to world society. These are the realities.

May the god(s) of the 4000 religions in this world save humanity. Amen.

"Today, the average Christian goes to church every week or so—shakes hands with a few Christian friends and says "God bless you"—listens to a gentle sermon and a few quiet hymns—then goes home feeling the "peace of God" in his heart. Because the Christian Church now conducts itself in a relatively civilized manner, a false-perception is created that religion has always been a tranquil force for good. That is not the case. Aside from the wholesale extermination of "witches," the Christian Church fought bitterly throughout its history—and is still fighting today—to impede scientific progress. Galileo, remember, was nearly put to death by the Church for constructing his telescope and discovering the moons of Jupiter." **– David Mills**

"Yes, I am an atheist. But just because I do not believe in your god does not mean I do not believe in anything. I believe in compassion, kindness, love, logic, equality, empathy, myself, integrity, honesty, and more." **– atheist quote**

"From the neurologic standpoint, I am simply lucky to harbor an innate and enduring neural fabric in my limbic lobe that is impervious to indoctrination enabling me to function usefully, and to develop ability, attitude and behavior of practical value in the society where I live without amalgamating them with religion and/or belief in supernatural." **– excerpt from "A Neurologist's Daring Escape from Steel Cage of Religion: A Long and Arduous Personal Journey to Reality" – Lazaro, R. Peppertree Press, 2022, Chapter 20**

ACKNOWLEDGMENT

The not-so-complimentary criticisms I received from my very religious classmates (class of 1970) about my negative stance on their belief system gave me the impetus to intellectualize religion and human behavior. I became broadminded, analytical, and sensible, enabling me to escape from the powerful grip of the Christian religion and to realize that good deeds and righteousness do not have to be amalgamated with belief in an invisible deity or with the existence of heaven and hell. I thank Dr. Alfredo I. Custodio, a staunch compatriot and classmate, the chief of the Grammar Police Force of our medical alumni group, and a successful physician-surgeon-writer living in the great state of Missouri for his candid and untainted criticisms. I affectionately call him the "Dave Barry" of our medical alumni group because of the uncanny similarities between his style of writing and that of Mr. Barry, a Pulitzer-winning humor columnist for Miami Herald. He is the author of "You've Got M@il.

BIBLIOGRAPHY

INTRODUCTION AND CHAPTER 1

Books

1. Adams, F. Origins of Existence, The Free Press, 2002

2. Sitchin, Z. The 12th Planet, Bear & Company, 1991

3. Lazaro, R. A Neurologist's Daring Escape from the Steel Cage of Religion: A long and arduous personal journey to reality. The Peppertree Press, 2022

Journal articles

1. Arzy, S, Idel,M, Landis, T, et al. (2005).Why revelations have occurred on mountains? Linking mystical experiences and cognitive neuroscience. Med Hypotheses. 65(5):841-845

2. Passie, T, Warncke, J. Peschel, et al. (2013). Neurotheology: neurobiological models of religious experience. Nervenarzt. 84(3):283-293

3. Sayadmansour, A. (2014).The relationship between brain and religion. Iran J Neurol. 13(1):52-55

Online sources

1. How Many Atheists Are There? /Psychology Today – www.psychologytoday.com/us/blog/the-secular-life/...

2. Most Atheist Countries 2022 – worldpopulationreview.com/…most-atheist-countries

3. When Did Homo Sapiens First Appear? – www.discovermagazine.com/planet-earth

4. Homo sapiens/The Smithsonian Institution's Human Origins – humanorigins.si.edu/…/species/homo-sapiens

5. Age of Earth – Wikipedia – en.wikipedia.org/wiki/Age _of_earth

6. WMAP –Age of the Universe – NASA - wmap.gsfc.nasa.gov/universe/uni_age.html

7. History of Sin: How it all began - www.scientificamerican.com/article/history-of...

8. sin/etymology, origin,and meaning of sin by etymonline – www.etymonline.com/word/Sin

9. The Origin of Sin - www.the gospelcoalition.org/essay/the-origin-of-sin

10. Seven deadly sins – en.wikipedia.org/wiki/Seven_deadly_sins

11. Sumerians – www.worldhistory.org/sumerians

12. The Sumerians – The True History of Ancient Civilizations – trueancienthistory.home.blog/…/02/26/the-sumerians

13. Sumerian religion – en.wikipedia.org/wiki/Sumerian_religion

14. Sodom and Gomorrah – en.wikipedia.org/wiki/Sodom_and_Gomorrah

15. Nineveh as Sin City – www.bibleodyssey.org/.../nineveh-as-sin-city

16. Origin of Religion – www.allaboutreligion.org/origin-of-religion.htm

17. History of religion – en.wikipedia.org/wiki/history_of_religion

Periodical

1. Kluger J, What Makes us Good/Evil. Time Magazine. Dec 3, 2007,53-60

CHAPTER 2

Book

1. Adams,RD, Victor,M, Principles of Neurology, McGraw-Hill, Inc., 1993

Journal articles

1. Koulousakis, P. Andrade, P, Visser-Vandewalle, et al. (2019). The Nucleus Basalis of Meynert and its Role in Deep Brain Stimulation for Cognitive Disorders: A Historical Perspective. J Alzheimers Dis. 69(4):905-919

2. Lee, MS, Rinne, JO, Marsden, CD. (2000). The pedunculopontine nucleus: its role in the genesis of movement disorders. Yonsei Med J. 41(2):167-184

3. Chinta, SJ, Anderson Jk. (2005). Dopaminergic Neurons. Int J Biochem Cell Biol. 37(5):942-946

4. Ranaldi, R. (2014). Dopamine and reward seeking: the role of ventral tegmental area. Rev Neurosci. 25(5):621-630

5. Wise RA, Jordan CJ. Dopamine, behavior and addiction (2021). J Biomed Sci. 28:83

6. Arias-Carrion, O, Stamelou, M, Murillo-Rodriguez, E, et al. Dopaminergic reward system: short integrative review. (2010). Int Arch Med. 3:10

7. Ross, A, Peselow, E. (2009). The neurobiology of addictive disorders. Clin Neuropharmacol. 32(5):269-276

8. Holly, EN, Miczek, KA. (2016). Ventral tegmental area dopamine revisited: effects of acute and repeated stress. Psychopharmacology (Berl). 233(2):163-186

9. Hornung, JP. (2003). The human raphe nuclei and the serotonergic system.26(4):331-343

10. Smythies J. (2005). The Cholinergic System. Int Rev Neurobiol. 64:1-122

11. Smythies J.(2005). The Norepinephrine System. Int Rev Neurobiol.64:173-211

12. Fulda S, Wetter TC (2005). Dopamine agonists for the treatment of restless legs syndrome. Expert Opin Pharmacother. 6(15):2655-2666

13. Mitchell, UH, Obray JD, Hunsaker E, et al. (2018). Peripheral Dopamine in Restless Legs Syndrome. Front Neurol. 9:155

14. Grotsch, P, Lange C, Wiesbeck GA, et al (2015). Pathological gambling induced by dopamine agonists: a case report. J Gambl Study. 31(1):295-297

15. Quickfall J, Suchowersky O. (2007). Pathological gambling associated with dopamine agonist use in restless legs syndrome. Parkinsonism Relat Disord. 13(8):535-536

16. Miller, NS, Ipeku R, Oberbamscheidt T. (2020). A Review of Cases of Marijuana and Violence. Int J Environ Res Public Health. 17(5):1578

17. Baumann, P. (1996). Pharmacokinetic-pharmacodynamics relationship of the selective serotonin re-uptake inhibitors. Clin Pharmacokinet. 3(6):444-469

18. Naglish, AC, Bozman, S, Brown ES, et al. (2019). Effect pf Selective Serotonin Reuptake Inhibitors on Healthcare Utilization in Patients with Post-Traumatic Stress Disorder and Alcohol Use Disorder. Alcohol Alcohol. 54(4):428-434

19. Van Heeringen, K, Mann, JJ. (2014). The neurobiology of suicide. Lancet Psychiatry. 1(1):63-72

20. Wislowska-Stanek, A, Kolosowska, K, Maciejak, P. (2021). Neurobiological basis of increased risk for suicidal behavior. 10(10):2519

21. Bach, H, Arango, V, Dwivedi, Y. (2012). Neuroanatomy of serotonergic abnormalities in suicide. editors. In: The neurobiological basis of suicide. Baton Raton (FL): CRC Press/Taylor & Francis; Chapter 2. Frontiers in Neuroscience

22. Barbui, A, Esposito, E, Cipriani, A. (2009). Selective serotonin reuptake inhibitors and risk of suicide: a systematic review of observational studies. CAMJ. 180(3):291-297

23. Karthik, S, Sharma, LP, Narayanaswamy J. (2020). Investigating the Role of Glutamate in Obsessive-Compulsive Disorder: Current Perspectives. Neuropsychiatr Dis Treat. 16:1003-1023

24. Tek, C, Ulug, B. (2001).Religiosity and religious obsessions in obsessive-compulsive disorders. Psychiatry Res. 1(104):99-108

25. Raphael, FJ, Rani, S, Ball, R, et al. (1996). Religion, ethnicity and obsessive-compulsive disorder. Int J Soc Psychiatry. 41(1): 38:44

26. Aouizerate, B, Guehl, D, Cuny, E, et al. (2004). Pathophysiology of obsessive compulsive disorder: a necessary link between phenomenology, neuropsychology, imaging, and physiology. Prog Neurobiol. 72(3): 195-221

27. Pittenger, C, Bloch, MH, Williams, K. (2011). Glutamate abnormalities in obsessive compulsive disorder: neurobiology, pathophysiology, and treatment. Pharmacol Ther. 132(3):314-332

28. Gadot, R, Najera,R, Hirani, S, et al. (2022). Efficacy of deep brain stimulation for treatment of resistant obsessive-compulsive disorder: systematic review and meta-analysis. J Neurol Neurosurg Psychiatry. 0:1-8. DOI:10.1136/jnnp-2021-328738

29. Jenike, MA. (1998). Neurosurgical treatment of obsessive-compulsive disorder. Br J Psychiatry. 35:79-90

30. Etherington, LA, Matthews, K, Akram, H. (2021). New Directions for Surgical Ablation Treatment of Obsessive Compulsive Disorder. Curr Top Behav Neurosci. 49:437-469

31. Luyten, L. (2020). The Bed Nucleus of the Stria Terminalis: Translational Deep Brain Stimulation to Reduce Anxiety. Neuroscientist. 26(3):278-284

32. Matthews, CA, Badner, JA, Andresen, JM, et al. (2012).Genome-wide linkage analysis of obsessive-compulsive disorder implicates chromosome 1p36. Biol Psychiatry. 72(8):629-636

33. Oumaya, M, Friedman, S, Pham, A, et al. (2008).Borderline personality disorder, self-mutilation and suicide: literature review.Encephale.34(5):452-458

34. Gordovez, FJ, McMahon, FJ. (2020). The genetics of bipolar disorder. Mol Psychiatry. 25(3):544-559

35. Craddock, N, Owen, M. (1994). Chromosomal aberration and bipolar disorder. Br J Psychiatry. 164(4):507-512

36. McCarthy, SE, Makarov, V, Kirov, G, et al.(2009). Microduplications of 6p11.2 are associated with Schizophrenia. Nat Genet. 41(11):1223-1227

37. Gejman, PV, Sanders, AR, Kendler, KS. (2011). Genetics of schizophrenia: New findings and challenges. Annu Rev Genomics and Hum Genet. 12:121-144

38. Distel, MA, Hottenga, JJ, Trull TJ. et al. (2008). Chromosome 9: Linkage for borderline personality disorder features. Psychiatr Genet. 18(6):302-307

39. Reichborn-Kjennerud T. (2010). Genetics of personality disorders. Clin Lab Med. 30(4):893-910

40. Ballard, C, Corbette, A. (2013). Agitation and aggression in people with Alzheimer's disease. Curr Opin Psychiatry. 20(3):252-259

41. Gallagher, D, Hermann, N. (2015). Agitation and aggression in Alzheimer's Disease: an update on pharmacological and psychosocial approaches to care. Neurodegener Dis Manag. 5(1):75-83

42. Devinsky, O, Lai, G. (2008). Spirituality and religion in epilepsy. Epilepsy Behav. 12(4):636-643

43. Tucker DM, Novelly, RA, Walker, PJ. (1987). Hyperreligiosity in temporal lobe epilepsy: redefining the relationship. J Nerv Ment Dis. 175(3):181-184

44. Garcia-Santaibanez, R, Sarva, H. (2015).Isolated Hyperreligiosity in a Patient with Temporal Lobe Epilepsy. Case Rep Neurol Med. 2015 Aug 13. Doi: 10.1155/2015/235856

45. Liu, Y, Tian, Y, Guo, R, et al. (2022). Anti-NMDA Receptor Encephalitis: Retrospective Analysis of 15 Cases, Literature Review, and implications for Gynecologists. J Health Eng. Mar 15;2022:4299791. Doi: 10.1155/2022/4299791

46. Bhavsar, V, Bhugra, D. (2008). Religious delusions: finding meanings in psychosis. Psychopathology. 41(3):165-172

47. Van Elk, Michiel, Aleman, A.(2017). Brain mechanisms in religion and spirituality: An integrative predictive processing framework. Neurosci Biobehav Rev. 73:359-378

48. Deeley, PQ. The religious brain (2004).Anthropol Med. 11(3):245-267

49. Tao,D, He,Z, Lin, Y, etal. (2021). Where does fear originate in the brain? A coordinate-based meta-analysis of explicit and implicit fear processing. Neuroimage. 15(227):117686. Doi: 10.1016/j.neuroimage.2020.117686

50. Pezze, MA, Feldon, J. (2004). Mesolimbic dopaminergic oathways in fear conditioning. Prog Neurobiol. 74(5):301-320

51. Garcia, R. (2017). Neurobiology of fear and specific phobias. Learn Mem. 24(9):462-471

52. Ohman, A, Carlsson,K, Lundquist, D, et al. (2007). On the unconscious subcortical origin of human fear. Physiol Behav. 92(1-2): 180-185

53. Ohman, A. (2005). The role of the amygdala in human fear: automatic detection of fear. Psychoneuroendocrinology. 30(10):953-958

54. Han, S, Ma,Y. (2014). Cultural differences in human brain activity. Neuroimage. 1(99):293-300

55. Gaw, AC.(2019). Religious Belief at the Level of the Brain: Neural Correlates and Influence of culture. J Nerv Ment Dis. 207(7):604-610

56. Carmona-Bayonas, A, Jimenez-Fonseca P, Olmos, CV, et al.(2017). Heperreligiosity in malignant brain tumors: a case report and accompanying bibliographic review. Neurocase. 23(1):88-95

57. Owen, AD, Hayward, RD, Koenig HG, et al.(2011). Religious factors and hippocampal atrophy in late life. PLOS ONE. 6(3):e17006. Doi: 10: 10.1371/journal.pone.0017006

58. Hayward, RD, Owen, AD, Koenig, HG, et al. (2011). Associations of religious behavior and experiences with extent of regional atrophy in the orbitofrontal cortex during older adulthood. Religion Brain Behav. 1(2):103-118

59. Ferguson, MA, Schaper, FLWVJ, Cohen, A, et al. (2022).A Neural Circuit for Spirituality and Religiosity Derived From Patients with Brain Lesions. Biological Psychiatry. 91(4):380-388

60. Mittersschiffthaler, MT, Ettinger, U, Mehta, M, et al (2006). Applications of functional magnetic resonance imaging in psychiatry. J Mag Reson Imaging. 23(6):851-861

61. Zipursky, RB, Meyer, JH, Verhoef, NP. (2007). PET and SPECT imaging in psychiatric disorders. Can J Psychiatry. 52(3):146-157

62. Nestadt, G, Grados, M, Samuels, JF. (2010). Genetics of OCD. Psychiatr Clin North Am. 33(1):141-158

63. Mahjani, B, Bey, K, Boberg, J, et al. (2021). Genetics of obsessive-compulsive disorder. Psychol Med. 51(13):2247-2259

Online sources

1. Kluver-Bucy syndrome – Wikipedia – en.wikipedia.org/wiki/kluver-Bucy_syndrome
2. Geschwind syndrome – Wikipedia – en.wikipedia.org/wiki/Geschwind_syndrome
3. Anti-NMDA Receptor Encephalitis – www.ncbi.nlm.gov/book/NBK551672
4. Religion and the brain. Dana Foundation – www.dana.org/article/religion-and-the-brain
5. Religious trauma syndrome – en-wikipedia.org/wiki/Religious_trauma_syndrome
6. Religious trauma syndrome – Journey Free – www.journeyfree.org/rts
7. Religious trauma – therapist.com/…identity-topics/religious-trauma
8. Neurotheology: How Science Can Enlighten Us…-Andrew Newberg – www.amazon.com/Neurotheology-Science-Enlighten
9. Andrew B. Newberg – en.wikipedia.org/wiki/Andrew_B_Newberg
10. Neuroanatomy, Substantia Nigra – www.ncbi.nih.gov/books/NBK536995
11. Wired to want? – bluewatercredit.com/wired-want-neuroscientists
12. Unexplained wealth of the Marcos family – en.wikipedia.org/wiki/unexplained_wealth_of_the…
13. Dopaminergic reward system: a short integrative review – PMC – www.ncbi.nlm.nih.gov.pmc/articles/PMC2958859
14. Religion and Dopamine addiction - dopamineproject.org/2011/07/religion-and …
15. Functional magnetic resonance imaging – en.wikipedia.org/wiki/functional_magnetic
16. Positron emission tomography of the brain – pubmed.ncbi.nlm.nih.gov/26447282

CHAPTER 3

Journal Articles

1. Raine A, Buschsbaum M, LaCasse L (1997). Brain abnormalities in murderers indicated by positron emission tomography. Biol Psychiatry. 42(6):495-508

2. Gavette , BE, Stern, RA, McKee, AC. (2011).Chronic Traumatic Encephalopathy: A Potential Late Effect of Sport-Related Concussive and Subconcussive Head Trauma. Clin Sports Med. 30:179-188

3. Williams, WH, Chitsabesan, P, Fazel S, et al. (2018) Traumatic Brain Injury" a potential cause of violent crime? Lancet Psychiatry. 5(10):836-844

4. Anckarsater H, Radovic, S, Svennerlind C, et al. (2009). Mental disorder is a cause of crime: the cornerstone of forensic psychiatry. Int J Law Psychiatry.32(6):342-347

5. Hodgins, S. (1992). Mental disorder, intellectual deficiency, and crime: Evidence from a birth cohort. Acrh Gen Psychiatry. 49(6)476-483

6. Cadoret, RJ, Leve, LD, Devor, E. (1997). Genetics of aggressive and violent behavior. Psychiatr Clin North Am. 20(2):301-322

7. Rolls ET.(2004). The function of the orbitofrontal cortex. Brain Cogn. 55(1):11-29

8. Rudebeck PH, Rich EL. (2018). Orbitofrontal cortex. Curr Biol. 28(18):R1083-R1088

9. Bao, AM, Swaab, DF. (2011).Sexual differentiation of the human brain:relation to gender identity, sexual orientation and neuropsychiatric disorders. Front Neuroendocrinol. 32(2):214-2126

10. Swaab, DF, Hofman MA. (1990). An enlarged suprachiasmatic nucleus in homosexual men. Brain Res. 557:141-148.

11. Savic, I, Berglund, H, Lindstrom, P. (2005). Brain response to putative pheromones in homosexual men. Proc Natl Acad Sc. USA. 102(20):7356-7361

12. Roselli, CE. (2018). Neurobiology of gender identity and sexual orientation. J Neuroendocrinol. 30(7):e1256. doi:10:1111/jne.12562

13. Swaab, DF, Wolff, SEC, Bao, AM. (2021). Sexual differentiation of the human hypothalamus: relationship to gender identity and sexual orientation. Handb Clin Neurol. 181:427-443

14. Abe, C, Johansson, E, Allzen, E, et al. (2014). Sexual orientation related differences in cortical thickness in males individuals. PLos One. 9(12):E114721

15. Anderson, NE, Harenski, KA. Harenski, CL, et al. (2019). Machine learning of gray matter differentiates sex in a large forensic sample. Human Brain Mapp. 40(5):1496-1506

16. Kinney III, RL. (2015). Homosexuality and scientific evidence: On suspect anecdotes, antiquated data, broad generalizations. Linacre Q. 82(4):362-390

17. Votinov, M, Goerlich, KS, Puiu AA, et al. (2021). Brain structure changes associated with sexual orientation. Sci Rep. doi.10.1038/s41598-021-84496-z

18. Van Moffaert, MM.(1990). Self-mutilation: diagnosis and practical treatment. Int J Psychiatry Med. 20(4):373-382

Online sources

1. Countries that criminalize homosexuality 2021 – www.statista.com/statistics/1227390

2. Seventy-one countries where homosexuality is illegal – www.newsweek.com/73 countries-where-its-illegal

3. Criminalization of homosexuality – en.wikipedia.org.wiki/Criminalization

4. People with Traumatic Brain Injuries More Likely to Commit Crimes – www.prisonlegalnews.org/news/2019/jun/3people

5. Traumatic brain injury – a potential cause of violent crime? – www.ncbi.nlm.nih.gov/pmc/articles/PMC6171742

6. Top 20 Notorious Cases of CTE – www.the sportster.com/entertainment/top-20

7. From Aaron Hernandez to Tyler Hilinski – www.oxygen.com/crime-time-who-may-have

8. Ex-NFL star Kellen Winslow committed crimes driven by CTE – www.usatoday.com/story/sports/nfl/2020/03/10/ex...

CHAPTER 4

Journal articles

1. Mendez, MS, Shapira, JS. (2011). Pedophile behavior from brain disease. J Sex Med. 8(4):1092-1100

2. Richer, M. Crismon, ML. (1993). Pharmacotherapy of sexual offenders. Ann Pharmacother. 27(3):316-320

3. Camperio, AS, Scarpazza C, Covelli, V, et al. (2019) Profiling acquired pedophilic behavior:Retrospective analysis of 66 Italian forensic cause of pedophilia. Int J Law Psychiatry. 67:101508

4. Schiffer, B, Peschel, T, Paul, T, et al (2007). Structural brain abnormalities in the frontostriatal system and cerebellum. J Psychiatr Res. 41(9):753-762

5. Alnemari, AM, Mansour, TR, Buehler, M, et al.(2016). Neural basis of pedophilia: altered sexual preference following traumatic brain injury. Int J Surg Case Rep. 25:221-224

6. Kneer, J, Borchardt, V, Kargel, C, et al. (2019). Diminished fronto-limbic functional connectivity in child sexual offenders. J, Psychiatr Res. 108:48-56

7. Fonteille, V, Redout, J, Lamothe, P, et al. (2019). Brain processing of pictures of children in men with pedophilic disorder: a positron emission tomography study. Neuroimage Clin. 21:101647

8. Schiltz, K, Witzel, J, Northoff, G,et al. (2007). Brain pathology in pedophilic offenders: evidence of volume reduction in the right amygdala and related diencephalic structures. Arch Gen Psychiatry. 64(6):737-746

9. Lopes, PMG, de Castro,CS, de Oliveira-Souza, R. (2020). The neurology of acquired pedophilia. Neurocase. 26(2):103-114

10. Tenbergen, G, Wittfoth, M, Frieling, H, et al. (2015). The neurobiology and psychology of pedophilia: Recent advances and challenges. 9:344

11. Schiffer, B, Krueger, T, Paul, T, et al. (2008). Brain response to visual sexual stimuli in homosexual pedophiles. J Psychiatry Neurosci. 33(1):23-33

12. Knott, V, Impey, D, Fisher, D, et al. (2016).Pedophilic brain potential responses to adult erotic stimuli. Brain Res. 1(1632):127-146

13. Fumagalli, M, Pravettoni, G. (2015). Pedophilia 30 years after brain injury. Neurol Sci. 36:481-482

14. Poeppl, TB, Nitschke, J, Santtila, P, et al. (2013). Association between brain structure and phenotypic characteristics in pedophilia. J Psychistr Res. 47(5):678-685

15. Simpson, G, Blaszczynski, A, Hodgkinson, A, (1990). Sex offending as a psychosocial sequel of traumatic brain injury. J Head Traum Rehab. 14(6):567-580

Online sources

1. Sexual abuse and the Catholic Church in the Philippines – www.alijazeera.com/features/2017/2016

2. 200 Filipino priests probed for sex scandals – www.philstar.com/headlines/2002/07/10/167762/200

3. Catholic Church sexual abuse cases by country – Wikipedia – en.wikipedia.org/wiki/Catholic _ Church_sexual

4. Timeline: Catholic Church sex abuse scandals – www.cnn/2017/06/29/world/time;ine-catholic

5. Paraphilia – Wikipedia – en.wikipedia.org/wiki/paraphilia

6. Roman Catholic Womenpriests – en.wikipedia.org/wiki/Roman_catholic_womenpriests

CHAPTER 5

Journal articles

1. Lent, R, Azevedo, FA, Andrade-Morales, CH, et al. (2012). How many neurons do you have? Some dogmas of quantitative neuroscience under revision. Eur J Neurosci. 35(1):1-9

2. Bahney, J, Von Bartheld, CS. (2018). The Cellular Composition and Glia-Neuron Ratio in the Spinal Cord of a Human and a Non-Human Primate: Comparison with other Species and Brain Regions. Anat Rec (Hoboken). 301(4):697-710

Online sources

1. Quotes about Heaven And Hell – www.quotemaster.org/Heaven+And+Hell

2. Soul –Wikipedia – en.wiki.org/wiki/Soul

3. Pope's Exorcist Says the Devil Is in the Vatican – abcnews.go.com/travel/chief-exorcist-rev

4. The centuries-old practice of exorcism is on the rise – www.news.vcu/article/The _centuriesold...

5. Exorcism and Spiritual Deliverance – insidethevatican.com/magazine/editorial/exorcism

6. Soul – Wikipedia – en.wikipedia.or.wiki/Soul
7. History of the location of the soul – en.wikipedia.org/wiki/History _of_the_location_of…
8. When did the concept of soul originate – profound-answers.com/when-did-the-concept-of…

CHAPTER 6

See journal articles cited in the text

CHAPTER 7

Online sources

1. Religiosity and intelligence – en.wikipedia.org/wiki/Religiosity _and_intelligence
2. The relation between intelligence and religiosity: a meta-analysis of 63 studies – pubmed.ncbi.nlm.nih.gov/23921675
3. Scrupulosity in the Confessional – Sanctuary Mental Health – Sanctuarymentalhealth.org/2021/10/22
4. Scrupulosity and confession – Catholic Archdiocese of Sydney – library.sydneycatholic.org/ask-a-priest/2017

CHAPTER 8

Online sources

1. Do Animals have Souls? – Outlawbiblestudent.org/do-animals –have-souls
2. Capital punishment – Wikipedia – en.wikipedia.org/wiki/Capital-punishment
3. The Difference Between Capital Punishment And Abortion – heidelblog.net/2018/01/the difference-abortion
4. When does a fetus have a heartbeat? – www.medicalnewstoday.com/articles/when-does-a...
5. First Fetal Movement – americanpregnancy.org/…/first-fetal-movement
6. Capital punishment – en.wikipedia.org/wiki/Capital_punishment
7. Capital punishment in Vatican City – en.wikipedia.org/wiki/Capital –punishment
8. Pope Francis: "death penalty inadmissible" – www.vaticannews.va/en/pope/news/2018/pope

CHAPTER 9

Books

1. Acharya, S. The Christ Conspiracy. The Greatest Story Ever Sold. Adventures Unlimited Press, 1999
2. Bushby, T. The Bible Fraud. The Pacific Blue Group, Inc., 2001
3. Leedom, TC. The Book Your Church Doesn't Want You To Read. Truth Seeker Books, 2003

Online sources

1. Anachronism – Wikipedia – en.wikipedia/org/wiki/anachronism
2. Christianity is an Anachronism/Ex Christian.Net – new.exchristian.net/2011/12christianity-is
3. A superb Article against Religious Indoctrination of Children – whyevolitionistrue.com/2020/14/a-superb
4. Indoctrination: The Good, The Bad and the Ugly – tacticalinvestor.com/indoctrination
5. Mark Twain Quotes on Religion – www.thoughtco.com/religion-quotes-by-mark-twain

CHAPTERS 10 AND 11

Journal articles

1. Champagne, FA. (2010). Early adversity and developmental outcomes. Perspect Psycho Sci. 5(5):564-574
2. Heijmans, BT, Tobi, EW, Stein, AD, et al. (2008). Persistent epigenetic differences associated with prenatal exposure to famine in humans. Proc Natl Acad Sci. 105(44):17046-17049
3. Lieneman, CC, Brabson, LA, Highlander, A, et al. (2017). Parent-child interaction therapy: current perspectives. Psychol Res Behav Manag. 10:239-256

4. Monk, C, Spicer, J, Champagne, FA. (2012). Linking prenatal maternal diversity to developmental outcomes in infants: The role of epigenetic pathways. Dev Psyhopathol. 24(4):1361-1376

5. Mulligan, CJ. (2016). Early environments, stress, and the epigenetics of human health. Annu Rev Anthropol. 45(1):233-249

6. Akiyama, T, Wakabayashi, S, Soma, A, et al.(2017). Epigenetic manipulation facilitates the generation of skeletal muscle cells from pluripotent stem cells. Stem Cells Int. 2017:7215010

7. Sharma S, Kelly T. (2010).Epigenetics in cancer. Carcinogenesis. 31(1):27-36

8. Husby, A. (2020). On the use of blood samples for screening DNA methylation in ecological epigenetic studies. Intgr Comp Biol. 60(6):1558-1566

9. Miao, C, Chang J. (2021). The important roles of microRNAs in depression: new research progress and future prospects. J Mol Med. (Berl). 99(5):619-636

10. Murphy, CP, Singewald, N. (2019). Role of microRNAs in anxiety and anxiety-related disorders. Curr Top Neurosci. 42:185-219

11. Rosa, JM, Formolo, DA, Yu, J, et al. (2022). The role of microRNA and microbiota in depression and anxiety. Front Behav Neurosci. 16:828258

12. Cadet, J, McCoy, MT, Jayanthi, S. (2016). Epigenetics and addiction. Clin Pharm Ther. 99(5):502-511

13. Nestler, EJ, Pena, CJ, Kundakovic, M, et al. (2016). Epigenetic basis of mental illness. The Neuroscientist. 22(5):447-463

14. Oberlander, TF, Weinberg,J, Papsdorf, M, et al. (2008). Prenatal exposure to maternal depression, neonatal methylation of human glucocorticoid receptor gene (NR3C1) and infant cortisol stress responses. Epigenetics. 3(2):97-106

15. Palmisano, M, Pandey, SC. (2017). Epigenetic mechanism of alcoholism and stress-related disorders. Alcohol. 60:7-18

16. Provencal, N, Binder, EB. (2015). The effects of early life stress on the epigenome: From the womb to adulthood and even before. Experimental Neurology. 268:10-20

17. Saavedra, K, Molina-Marquez, AM, Saavedra N, et al. (2016). Epigenetic modifications of major depressive disorder. Int J Mol Sci. 17(8):1279

18. Zhang, H, Gelernter, J. (2017). DNA methylation and alcohol use disorders; Progress and challenges. Am J Addict. 26(5):502-515

19. Vandermeers, F, Sriramareddy, SN, Costa, C, et al. (2013). The role of epigenetics in malignant pleural mesothelioma. Lung Cancer. 8(3):311-318

20. Jones, PA, Ohtani, H, Chakravarthy A, et al. (2019). Epigenetic therapy in immune-oncology. Nature. 19:151-161

21. Kumsta,R. (2019). The role of epigenetics for understanding mental health difficulties and its implications for psychotherapy research. Pscyhol Psychother. 92(2):190-207

22. Kruger, TGC, Sinke, C, Knee, J, et al. (2019).Child sexual offenders show prenatal an epigenetic alterations of the androgen system.9(1):28

23. Cole, J, Morris, P, Dickman, MS, et al. (2016). The therapeutic potential of epigenetic manipulation during infectious diseases. Pharmacol Ther. 167:85-99

24. Jahn, K, Kurz, B, Sinke, C, et al. (2022). Serotonin system-associated genetic and epigenetic change in pedophilic and child sexual offending. J Psychiatr Res. 145:60-69

25. Chuang, JC, Jones, PA. (2007). Epigenetics and microRNAs. Ped Res. 61(5 pt2):24R-29R

26. Rice, WR, Friberg, U, Gavrilets, S.(2012). Homosexuality as a consequence of epigenetically canalized sexual development. Q Rev Biol. 87(4):343-368.

27. Ngun, TC, Villain, E. (2014). The biological basis of human sexual orientation: is there a role for epigenetics? Adv Genet. 86:167-84

28. Macke, JP, Hu, N, Hu, S, et al (1993). Sequence variation in the androgen receptor gene is not a common determinant of male orientation. Am J Hum Genet. 53(4):844-852

29. Ford, G, Macgregor A, Miot S. (2013). Nanopsychiatry – the potential role of nanotechnologies in the future of psychiatry: a systematic review. Eur Neuropsychopharmacol. 9:1067-1071

30. Sobarzo-Sanchez, E, Nabavi, SM, Uriarta, E, et al.(2015). Nanoparticles in the treatment of mental disorders: a new tool in the psychiatric medication. Curr Top Med Chem. 15(4):282-286

31. Chhabra, R, Tosi, G, Grabrucker, AM. (2015). Emerging use of nanotechnology in the treatment of neurological disorders. Curr Pharm Des. 21(22):3111-3130

32. Jorgensen, RA. (2011). Epigenetics: Biology's Quantum Mechanics. Front Plant Sci. Apr 12;2:10

33. Rees, CA, Lee, LK, Fleegler, EW, et al.(2019). Mass School Shootings in the United States: A Novel Root Cause Analysis Using Lay Press Reports. Clin Pediatr (Phila). 58(13);1423-1428

34. Towers, S, Gomez-Lievano, A, Khan, M. et al. (2015).Contagion in Mass Killings and School Shootings. PLos One. 10(7):e0117259. Doi: 10:1371/journal.pone.0117259.

Online source

1. History of Epigenetics: Johns Hopkins Kimmel Cancer Center – www.hopkinsmedicine.org/...epigenetics/history.html

2. A Brief History of Epigenetics –PMC – www.ncbi.nlm.gov/PMC3941222

3. SUMO protein – en.wikipedia.org/wiki/SUMO_protein

4. Histone modification – an overview – www.sciencedirect.com/.../histone-modification

5. Epigenetics: Why Identical Twins Are Not Really Identical – www/scienceprofonline.com/genetics/epigenetics

6. Identical Twins are Living Epigenetic Experiments – The Atlantic – www.theatlantic.com/.../05/twin-epigenetics/560189

7. Effect of Epigenetic Differences in Identical Twins - link.springer.com/referenceworkentry/10.1007/978

8. List of school shootings in the United States – en.wikipedia.org/wiki/List_of_school _shootings_in…

9. A list of Recent Mass Shootings in the United States – www.nytimes.com/2021/03/23/us/us-mass-shootings.html

10. Mental illness, Mass Shootings and the Future of Psychiatric – www.ncbi.nlm.gov/pmc/articles/PMC7803479

11. The Psychology Behind Mass Shootings – whywesuffer.com/the-psychology-behind-mass-shootings

12. Can epigenetics explain homosexuality puzzle? – https://www.science.org/doi/full/10.1126/science.350.8257.148

13. Epigenetic theories of homosexuality – en.wikipedia.org/wiki/Epigenetic_theories_of…

14. Behavioral epigenetics – www.ncbi.nlm.gov/omc/articles/PMC3783959

15. Epigenetic Inheritance: Concepts, Mechanisms and Perspectives – www.ncbi.nlm.nih.gov/pmc/articles/PMC6172332

16. Quantum mechanics – en .wikipedia/org/wiki/quantum_mechanics

17. What is Quantum Physics – scienceexchange.caltech.edu/…quantum-physics

Art works provided by Maa Illustrations, art@maaillustrations.com

Made in the USA
Monee, IL
03 November 2026

67378725R10063